VICTORY OVER SICKLE CELL:

IGNITING VIBRANT HEALTH

&

INSPIRING TRANSFORMATION

HASINA IRELAND
RMT, RHN

DISCLAIMER

This book is a comprehensive resource, drawing from Hasina Ireland's vast professional expertise and personal experiences. It includes some of her original poetry, created over the years as a means of expressing emotions and navigating life's challenges, which seamlessly intertwine with the topics discussed.

The information presented here is intended for educational purposes only. It is not a substitute for professional medical advice or treatment. Readers are advised not to alter or delay any medical therapy prescribed by a qualified healthcare provider. It is essential to consult with a healthcare professional regarding health-related concerns and decisions.

Hasina shows she's a warrior. Having the strength to battle sickle cell and be an advocate for superior health. This book shows her depths and triumphs. I picked up some great tips for better health from this book, and I'd definitely suggest checking out her amazing services too.

Emilee "Emergy" B.

****

From the tender age of three months, Hasina has endured immense pain caused by sickle cell disease. As an adult, she turned to holistic nutrition, educating herself and using her knowledge to help others facing similar struggles and stigmas. Her devotion to holistic healing extends beyond herself—she radiates strength, courage, determination, and an uplifting energy that inspires those around her.

I also love how she combines professionalism with a warm, engaging style that draws readers into her journey. Through heartfelt quotes, personal reflections, practical guidance, and phenomenal poetry, she creates an experience that is both informative and deeply moving. Her book is a testament to resilience and a celebration of life despite challenges.

Sandra O'Reggio

Sickle Cell Warrior Advocate/Supporter

****

"A whole new perspective will awaken your enthusiasm for life." - Hasina Ireland.

A potent health book that everyone will absolutely benefit from reading. An eye-opening look at a holistic health journey. With added artistic expression of poetry as a strong bonus, Hasina shares her powerful testimony of how she maneuvers through life as a sickle cell warrior. From the stage of learning about what sickle cell is and how it affects her body, all the way to the point of teaching others how to understand and maximize their own unique body capabilities. This book will inspire you to take better care of yourself the natural way, through cell food and healthy practices. The difference between listening and understanding your own body, rather than relying on the recommendation of pharmaceutical drugs.

Kirk Ireland

Sickle Cell Warrior Advocate/Supporter

****

Through extensive research and a lifetime of personal battles, the author emerges as a true warrior in search of healing and peace. This book offers a rare insight into sickle cell anemia, blending lived experience with holistic approaches to health and nutrition.

More than just a guide on managing sickle cell, it's an eye-opening journey that teaches readers how to harness the body's natural power to heal. No matter your age, background, or health status, this book encourages a fresh approach to life. The details within have boosted my endurance, mental health, and energy, inspiring a lifestyle rooted in balance, wellness, and self-empowerment.

Yuwii

Athlete/Entertainer

Dedication

For every dreamer with a vision, every fighter with a scar, and every believer with hope—may you rise with strength, thrive with wellness, and live with unstoppable vitality.

Acknowledgment

Behind the creation of this book are incredible individuals who have supported me, both directly and indirectly, throughout my journey living with sickle cell anemia. To everyone who has contributed to the advocacy and awareness of this condition, your efforts are deeply appreciated.

I am profoundly grateful for the universal forces that have guided and protected me, especially during moments of despair.

Special thanks to my amazing mother, Sandra, and brother, Kirk. Your unwavering support during some of my toughest times has been vital and indispensable. To all who visited me, whether at home or in the hospital, during my health challenges, your presence was a tremendous source of comfort. To my father, sister Sade, and nephew Erick, I extend many blessings.

To my son Unaz, you are my sunshine and superstar. You bring unparalleled joy into my life. I love and cherish you with all my heart.

Mama, your wise words, "Wos dan many, betta dan plenty," have been a source of strength during difficult times. One day at a time. Continue Resting in Power. You have been one of the strongest women I've known, and I'm so grateful for your love and confidence in me.

I also extend my gratitude to my instructors and coaches for their knowledge, patience, and willingness to share their expertise in personal development, holistic nutrition, Reiki, metaphysics, phlebotomy, pathophysiology, biology, massage therapy, and life itself.

Jessica, thank you for hiring me at Garlic Grove in 1999, where my health journey truly began.

Lastly, thank you to all the caring nurses, physicians, and specialists who have worked with me over the years. Your dedication to my care during follow-up appointments, routine procedures, and hospital admissions has been exceptional.

It is my pleasure to share my experience and journey on sickle cell anemia with you. Through education, practical applications, and spoken word, I hope this book provides value and insight. Thank you, reader, for choosing this book.

Contents

About the Author

Hasina is deeply committed to helping others achieve long-term wellness through scientific, practical, and proven information and therapeutic assistance. With a diverse background in nutrition, Reiki, phlebotomy, and massage therapy, she has been dedicated to her practice since 2005. Her expertise centers on improving organ health and identifying imbalances that hinder the body's natural healing processes.

Understanding the profound physical, emotional, mental, and spiritual challenges her clients face, Hasina creates individualized plans that address their primary concerns. She then helps them set realistic goals and provides focused guidance to achieve these objectives. Her approach is both compassionate and evidence-based, ensuring that each client receives tailored support for their unique needs.

In her personal journey, Hasina finds balance and inspiration through spoken word, yoga, and connecting with nature. Overcoming her own health challenges has deepened her dedication to promoting a healthier, happier life for herself and her clients. She firmly believes that life is a blessing and that protecting one's health is paramount.

Feel free to contact **Essential Healing** *for more information on any of the methods discussed to improve the health of your cells, tissues, organs, and overall health.*

Visit www.essentialhealingsolutions.ca/ for your wellness options.

Chapter 1
Managing Sickle Cell: Take Charge, Live Strong

When I first met Shauna, she was a single mother of three daughters, working a typical 9-5 job and doing her best to maintain the most fulfilling life possible for herself and her family. This was despite facing moments where she was sidelined by sharp, stabbing pain and frequent sickle cell episodes. At that time, she had been with her employer for five years, and they had been very accommodating when she needed to call in sick or take time off.

Feeling progressively emptier and with her episodes growing more intense, she eventually had a breakdown, and her body completely crashed. Escorted to the hospital once again, Shauna felt incapable of providing for her daughters, Bonnet, Gloria, and Amanda. At the time, she couldn't manage even the simplest tasks on her own, such as making it to the washroom, taking a shower, or even brushing her teeth. The inability to move with ease hit her hard.

She overheard Bonnet, her youngest, speaking softly to her sister Amanda, "It's scary when Mommy has to stay in the hospital… sometimes I think she might not come home."

Hearing this was deeply disheartening for Shauna. She felt that both her life and her daughters' lives were at stake if she didn't take control and find a way to make things better.

If not her, then who?

Spending a week in the hospital multiple times a year had given her plenty of time to think, and this wasn't the first instance where she'd had thoughts like this. But this time was different.

This time, she felt the urge to once and for all take it upon herself to do something out of the ordinary. To prove to herself and her family that things would be okay. Not just through hopeful, wishful thinking, but by real actions, actual facts, and visible results.

How could this happen? She had no idea. As a mother, Shauna had little time for herself, or perhaps it's better to say, *she chose not to take time for herself* because she felt it would be selfish. Lying down for a nap when she felt she needed to rest didn't seem fair to her daughters. What she realized in her hospital bed was that it wasn't fair to herself either, nor to them, to see her in such pain and so much calamity, so often. She knew she had to do something. This was costing her far more than time. It was costing her joy, her sanity, and her family's mental and emotional well-being, too. Even though she was only in her late 40s, she was dealing with crippling symptoms that made her feel as if she were about to leave this earth.

****

<u>Temporary Residence</u>

This is but a temporary residence

Comprised of the fake and material things

That fill the heart and mind with no relevance

No benevolence

All but a mist of time tryin' to find somethin' to call,

Mine

No, it ain't all just fine

For our physical existence can suddenly get snatched

So don't get too attached and believe the world

In all its robotic fallacies and superstitions

Cease flirting with danger and follow the true path

To complete your mission

Listen...

Our goal is to select the road

Taking us away from the black hole so we can abstain

From the simple desires that war against our souls

Control

Dissect your intellect and dispose of unnecessary pain

That strains the brain in vain

Moral bankruptcies on the rise

Peace dies

Hate and slander of the wise

Ain't no surprise exchanging truth for lies

We're truly living amongst the evil reign

Some struggling to remain sane

And others absorbed in this daze

In this phase, exit the maze

Eradicate useless ways and enter into the place

Of humility and eternity

In these last days

Seeds scattered amongst the path, the thorns

And rocky places rather than good soil

Having the message snatched away, having no root

And being unfruitful

This mostly being rejected than accepted

But remember that this is but a temporary residence

We are brave slaves living our lives in rhythmic waves

Sometimes up, sometimes down, and

Sometimes, finding ourselves flowing round and round

Who, me?

I'm learning to stand firm

Knowing that my Divine Source uttered

"Many are the plans in a man's heart, but it is the Lord's purpose that prevails."

Therefore, my character entails

Peace, truth, and love

A desire to heal and be healed

A spirit of hope

Patient in tribulation

And seeking to receive my complete emancipation

And though I am blessed with the breath of life

I am dead amongst this world of strife

Governments running things like

Conspiracy, monopoly, hypocrisy,

All a blasphemy living in this land of sovereignty

Take the time to pause and reflect

The direct neglect of respect

Intersect and let the word be heard

Apply these lessons daily with power

Beware, keep watch, and stand on guard

For we do not know the day

Nor the hour

For this is but a temporary residence

****

Cry For Help

No. That's it. Enough is enough, she thought. *If not now, then when? Is there another way?* In her drugged-out daze, as the IV replenished her fluids and high doses of medication worked to dull the pain, she wondered if she would ever be able to conquer the negative emotions that came with living with this condition.

She was in such a trance that it felt like she almost had nothing to lose. She had to do this for herself. Her daughters depended on her. She had to discover a way not only to reduce the number of hospital visits, but also to reduce the intensity and frequency of those life-sucking episodes. For many years, she had been struggling to manage her sickle cell while running her household, and it had never been easy. But sometimes "rock bottom" is exactly where you need to be before you're forced to make a change. That was definitely what happened to Shauna.

She knew she wasn't going anywhere anytime soon. Bed rest with massive discomfort was all too familiar, and remembering other similar episodes left her feeling both upset and sad simultaneously.

What is this? she thought. Then it came to her. Her eyes widened as her thoughts suddenly were in a state of revival.

What doesn't kill you makes you stronger, that was her next thought. But no... sickle cell has the potential to shorten your lifespan, damage your organs, and even take your life. That saying did not do her justice. Even so, she is still a warrior.

She did not feel strong at that moment. She was in a hospital bed and would be there for another few days or so. Yet, right then and there, she made a promise to herself: She would do her best, if it took everything she had, to avoid returning to the hospital. Yes, it was the one place that could save her from agony and complications, but it also sucked the life out of her.

****

<u>*Drained*</u>

My soul is screaming effortlessly

Yet nothing is deemed unwritten

I struggle to listen defenselessly

For my mind hinders thinkin'

All day, my body feels too weak

Though I am able to survive

Life for me is unbelievably bleak

That's enough to be deprived

Too many tears are overflowing

They cannot be held back

My heartbeat skips unknowing

Too many good emotions, I lack

Night and day, I deeply yearn

For things to fit together

Ultimately, I know I must learn

I can't let this go on forever

What can I do to reassure myself

That this is all life's miracle process?

Confusion is multiplying itself

Only time can release this mess

Sure enough, I can unlock my abstained door

But where do I turn to find the key?

****

I've been hospitalized far too many times to count, and I know the frustrations that come along with this debilitating condition. It is because I can relate to stories like Shauna's that I am so committed to educating and facilitating individuals like her towards the health and wellness they so truly deserve. The best way to initiate permanent change is to deeply feel why change is needed, and sometimes, these painful, soul-wrenching experiences are what it takes to accomplish this.

Meeting Shauna

While Shauna lay in a hospital bed, asking herself how she could manage her sickle cell without feeling sick all the time, she had no idea she was launching us both on a personal, professional, and scientific journey.

Many specialists give recommendations that may be valid, but they often come with inconsistencies and tremendous amounts of side effects. My interest lies in helping individuals prevent the episodes that land them in the hospital in the first place.

On this particular day, I was discussing preventative measures with a client dealing with chronic pain. He mentioned that he and his wife were looking after his cousin Shauna's three daughters, as she was currently in the hospital, admitted with an acute crisis. I asked for permission to speak with her. We ended up talking the next day, and I was able to visit her the day after that.

Being in a hospital still brings anxiety to me, remembering the many times I entered those doors in such a dreadful state, having to be jabbed time and time again to find my tiny veins that tend to collapse easily. As I entered her room, our eyes met, and in those few seconds, it was almost as if we had a conversation. In her eyes, I could see it all, the despair, the weakness, the cry for help, the vulnerability.

We ended up talking for hours. We laughed, we cried, we shared similar experiences and emotional ups and downs related to sickle cell. She mentioned that she had been offered a promotion at her company that would increase her income, allowing her to spend more time with her children, and giving her the opportunity to hire and educate other employees. It was a great opportunity, but she hesitated to take it because she feared it would affect her health due to the stress of additional responsibilities, or that her health would interfere with the job if she needed time off.

One of the many characteristics that gets magnified for sickle cell patients is fear. "What if I get sick?" And yes, for many activities and decisions we make, we obviously have to consider our condition. On the other hand, that fear can keep us back from pursuing our passions and our calling. Living with sickle cell shouldn't hold you back in anything. Know your limits, yes. Be too careful, no.

Shauna avoided doing many things, making her so resentful and drained that it created a deficiency in her motivation and in the vital life force of both her body and mind. This time was different. This time, she wanted to make a change for good. She was ready and willing. It came down to a choice: continue in the downward cycle she was in or create the life she desired for herself and her daughters. She didn't want to feel like a burden, and she wanted her daughters to see that she was capable of making a change.

It was only up to one person, and that was herself. It was evident that Shauna understood the options given by her doctors, but she didn't want to go with just any recommendation they threw at her because of her negative encounters in the past.

As I learned more about Shauna and her situation, it closely mirrored certain aspects of my own experiences. Her despair challenged her to uncover an unwavering drive to seek another path for her healing and the will to make a difference in her own life.

The same as it did mine.

****

<u>I Need To Be Free</u>

I want to be free

And use the right key for my presented opportunity

Trying to dispel influential hostility

Scaring my conscience and eating away at the cause

I need to pause

Meditate on the reason of this season

In strength, courage, and dedication

The battle in my mind has got to be overcome

Dismantled, disfigured, and done

Won by the battles of my beating heart

There's pounding, there's pounding

There's pounding memories and illusions

Of situations beyond my control

Wrapped around the matter with a tight grip and hold

I need to unfold the…

Disharmony, despondency, animosity, atrocity, self-pity

And lack of awareness within each step I take

There's too many issues holding me down

Now, attempting to conquer the process

Between birth and death

My flesh desires to win the game

It can be so unjust, selfish, ignorant, and profane

Leaving only I to blame

What a shame

Continue to guide me in the path of righteousness I pray

And day by day

I slay evil away

So, in this way, I will break free

I want to be

Free from the bars that hold my scars

Slowly healing wounds that I am still feeling

From the history of my being, seeing

Disappointed faces from my past troubled cases

Oh, total body compression within these learning sessions

I am trapped alone in my confusion

In attempt to seek my own solution

But thanks to the love of my lifeline

I realize the heights that I must climb

In time

In time comes the answer, the wisdom, the growth

I've learned to bear the weight

Of fear, heartache, pain and rejection

A whole selection of

Open sores and hidden doors

I need that divine connection

The correction held hostage inside of me

I need to be free

Chapter 2
My Journey Through Pain:
Finding Strength in the Struggle

I was born in Montreal in 1981, weighing 5 pounds 13 ounces. "Hello world, here I am!" I was pretty small, but considered healthy with no obvious health problems. But three months later, in January 1982, my world changed. My hands and feet began to swell. I was in pain, though the only way I could show it was through constant, unusually intense irritability – more than usual. My mother sensed something was terribly wrong as my screams and cries didn't stop. Worried and confused, she took me to the hospital, where my parents discovered I was experiencing my first sickle cell crisis.

What?! Sickle cell? Neither of my parents had ever heard of it before. This diagnosis came as a total shock. In time, they learned how I inherited the genetic mutation, and what they could do to help me live as healthy a life as possible, despite the symptoms and complications my sickle-shaped cells would bring over the years.

Doctors advised my mother to pay close attention whenever I cried. She was told to gently squeeze me from head to toe, and wherever I screamed the most, that's where I was having pain. Most of the time, she already knew the areas affected due to swelling (for example, my hands or feet). I was admitted regularly to Montreal Children's Hospital, where I received IV treatments infused with codeine. Because my veins were so difficult to access, the decision was made to shave a small patch of my head and insert the IV there. Other times, they managed to insert the IV into a vein in my hand or foot. I could only imagine what my parents were going through at that time.

I was routinely admitted to the hospital approximately six times per year, often staying for up to seven days. I would receive daily folic acid and codeine to manage the frequent episodes I was experiencing. This later progressed to other strong pain medications as an adult, such as Demerol, Morphine, and Oxycodone. When I was about seven years old, my family moved to Toronto. By then, going back and forth to the hospital became routine.

****

<u>*Darkness*</u>

It feels like I'm drowning, but there's no water surrounding me

It could be the tears flowing from my eyes

Catching up so suddenly

For this, my body is drained from all grateful reality

Which is why I see no reason to live on, joyful and happily

I wonder if my mind could pound any harder

Or if my insides could scream any louder

It's clear to state that this hurtful process won't drift any faster

Since my thundering heartbeat is fading away softer and softer

****

More than once, doctors recommended that I receive a blood transfusion. Researchers and physicians also suggested enrolling me in a trial for the drug hydroxyurea, which is now widely used for patients with sickle cell. My parents refused both options. My father preferred natural methods and limited medical interventions as much as possible. This may have influenced my own tendency towards holistic health care methods in the years that followed.

Physicians advised my parents to keep me warm and to steer me away from activities that required too much energy. I remember wanting to do gymnastics, but I was told it would be too much for me. I enjoyed triple jump, skating, and volleyball, but none of them lasted because I couldn't keep up with my participation in them. The triple jump sometimes knocked the wind out of me, the skating rinks were too cold, and volleyball hurt my wrists, often triggering painful episodes. So, I just paid attention to academics instead. My schoolwork was always with me at my hospital bedside. The need to catch up was a constant theme throughout elementary school, middle school, high school, and well into adulthood.

My Decision To Seek Natural Means

Regularly feeling groggy from medications and weak from recovering sparked further interest in holistic health. In about grade 10 or so, gallstones ended up being one of the final straws. My doctor mentioned that this is a common complication of sickle cell, but at the time, I had no idea what was going on. At first, my doctor just said to take Tums. This helped with the pain after eating, but then I started to feel the discomfort more often. This went on for weeks until I ended up back at Sick Kids Hospital (literally my second home at the time). There, I was advised to have my gallbladder removed, so I did.

When I was in a high school co-op program, where we would spend time working in a business to help with learning about an occupation we wanted to pursue, I had no idea what field of health I should get into. Health and wellness were (and still are) my interests. Then it dawned on me that I should take responsibility for my own health. I decided to work in a health food store. Mind you, I had never set foot in one until then. Other than previous visits to Jamaica, where my grandmother provided us with healing herbs and concoctions to drink as a child, I never really questioned it. That was just something we had to do. Circling back to the health food store, being introduced to the world of herbs, vitamins, minerals, and supplements opened a whole new perspective to me.

Reading through a reference book in the store one day, I stumbled across a natural technique to get rid of gallstones, called a gallbladder flush. I was surprised and disappointed at the same time. Disappointed that I didn't know options like these existed. It just demonstrates that if you seek, you shall find, but everyone is uniquely different, so please speak with your health care provider before trying anything new.

Most physicians would not recommend trying out methods like this, but what if I'd known about that option? I'm sure I would have tried it out, instead of being cut open and having my organ stripped from my body. It was a common procedure, the doctor told me, and yes, the body can function fine without a gallbladder. That may be so, but we are all born with one. There's a reason it's a part of our physiology, whether we can function without it or not.

I continued to develop more interest in esoteric, metaphysical, and energetic practices. I was amazed at what I was learning, like how every organ not only had a specific function, but also corresponded to various energy centers within us, ultimately affecting our thoughts, emotions, and actions. Tapping into the organs that had been affected by harsh medications over the years proved to be beneficial for me. For example, I care for my liver by eating to support that organ and taking whole food supplements. I also pay close attention to my emotions because certain emotions, like anger, are associated with the liver. I continuously address both my physical and emotional needs with my personal holistic program.

There's an accumulation of past traumas in all realms that has infiltrated my cellular core, but as long as I can recognize them and chip away at the damage to move forward, that's all that matters. Hopefully, you feel the same in your own situation. Because I know how traumatic sickle cell can be on its own, life can make things just a bit more challenging, which contributes to us referring to ourselves as sickle cell warriors. Rightfully so.

After graduating from high school, I worked in the same health food store for about six years. I decided to learn Reiki, which is a restorative technique using the universal life force energy that flows through all living things. Gravitating to and becoming aware of energetic healing in my teenage years was intensified after learning more about how nutrients can affect our every being. The designation of Reiki Level I in the year 2000 was earned by working with a Master Reiki teacher of the Usui method. In 2001, I graduated from the

Canadian School of Natural Nutrition as a registered holistic nutritionist. Two months later, I gave birth to my son.

****

<u>*Mutual Connection*</u>

Do not underestimate the creation

Of a man and a woman

I will begin to express my best on masculinity

Naw, I ain't talkin' 'bout the process of meiosis

Making those x – y chromosomes

Shaping the genetic blueprint of DNA

Hey

This is my interpretation of a man that's whole and true

Dedicated, respectful, courageous, faithful, proactive

Conscious and real in all that he can do

He is guided by the divine spirits

Of exceptional wisdom from ancient times

Living his life in the struggles of this world, yet

Able to maintain a mighty mind

Using his strength to uplift his kind

22

His heart so profound – eyes majestic, burin' like fire and

Personal desires radiating

For passionate upliftment, persistent movements

And powerful achievements

He is a seed-bearing fruit

Not just one of those working in this system

With a tie and suit

No flashing around his loot

For soul-killing material things

Only concerned with what is necessary

Oh, and if he decides to find a mate

She will be no bait for him to simply enter her gate

This is a woman

The womb of mankind

An intellectual educator

An example of self-control

Creative, a nurturer, and firm from mind to body to soul

She is a Queen of her domain

Having ancient divinity circulating through her veins

And like the energy that gives us light

She is the manifestation that simply keeps giving

Giving hope, knowledge, comfort, strength, health,

Direction and affection wholeheartedly

Great is she in the spirit of our universal intelligence

Not to prove but to serve amongst this learning curve

And what has been found

Is that she must remain on solid ground

For the success and growth of our society

Now when this man and this woman unite

Great expectations are conceived

Spiritual fixation like a lock and key

Mental clarity

And a physical relation as good as it can be

May result in a new birth

Worth universal appreciation

A gift of divine power aligned on that latitude

Where, together, the practice

Is an attitude of gratitude

Contented to just be and to complement each other freely

Completely, effortlessly in monogamy

Sharing a humble journey as sweet as honey

That portrays life like a vast expanse

The meditations of you and me

Enlightening their union to higher heights

Working their family with a foundation so opulent

Filled with purpose

And a virtue so meaningful that their path is unstoppable

The creation of a man and a woman

Is not simply meant to be

Be hypnotized by the word 'love'

Be self-absorbed in empty acts of indulgence

But to be at each other's mercy

Thirsty for the now, and having the satisfaction

Of individualized perfection

Within their mutual connection

****

My Son Was Born

I was so excited, and yet worried at the same time. I did not want my son to have to go through the same difficulties I've had to. His father was tested and discovered he is a carrier of the sickle cell gene (hemoglobin SC), so he has the potential to pass on the gene. Since I was diagnosed with SS (Hb SS is considered a more severe form of sickle cell disease), the chances of my son having SS were 50-50. That was huge.

I knew it had to do with genetics, but at the same time, I knew the power of words through prayer and how strong emotion can enhance this power. I knew this had the force to heal and the power to reduce the chances of my son receiving the diagnosis of SS. Over time, I had the true belief that he would be okay, and thankfully, my prayers were answered.

My high-risk pregnancy went full-term with no serious complications, other than my staying in the hospital for about a week before his delivery. Labor and delivery were another story. Okay, long story short – two days in labor, two epidurals, both of which did not help much for the pain, and an emergency cesarean section. Besides that, all turned out well, fortunately.

****

<u>***My Son Is Here***</u>

My son is here, near my bedside

Satisfied with pride, I

Sit back and compose

These lines my heart chose

Froze

Time froze

Looking at your precious

Beloved body

I am enchanted

Granted with a beauty so gracious

Your face just – lightens the room

My womb

It carried you throughout

Now you're out - here with me

Mommy is what you will speak

Unique is your physique

So unbelievable you are

The atmosphere is clear

My son is finally here

****

I was blessed to give birth to a healthy baby and get through pregnancy with absolutely no episodes and childbirth with no major complications. Over the years, my son has seen me go through such intense episodes that I wish he hadn't had to experience. I know it has made him stronger in many aspects as a person. He also knows what the consequences could be if his partner or child is affected. It is possible for him to pass on the gene as a carrier, though his experience with me has equipped him well for making his own informed decision.

PURSUING MY INTEREST

With what I'd been living with, it was a natural progression for me to continue my journey in the health field by participating in workshops, courses, programs, and offering services and techniques that help prevent or mitigate pain. By experimenting with different therapies and professional-grade supplements, I have so far been able to gradually reduce my hospital admissions from up to 6 admissions per year to absolutely zero in 2019-2024. This is a huge accomplishment. I feel the change. I see the change. I feel it in my soul. Progress is continuing over time with shorter durations of episodes experienced, and I am able to manage well at home with help from my mom, brother, and son. I've been truly blessed by their support, and I would love to see ample assistance for those in need who may not be so fortunate. With the help of sickle cell organizations and associations, there should be no reason for you to be suffering alone.

Writing and the spoken word have enabled me to express my emotions to proceed through my journey. My background in energy therapy, holistic nutrition, phlebotomy, and massage therapy has brought new knowledge, which I know has improved my condition. So, there is no reason for me to keep what I know to myself. Learning from trial and error and seeing the benefits and improvement over time with myself and clients has brought me to the place I am now – writing this book. I can now share what I've learned because there has been not only scientific proof, but also practical proof.

The functions of our true essential self go beyond what we can understand with our conscious mind. When we surrender to this, we can see the important role it plays in our well-being, a fact that is ignored by many. If we never had any challenges, then how would we grow? My experiences have been fueled by the work I've done to build my strength and my cells while also identifying the areas I need to focus on for effective recovery, taking preventative measures, and sharing the methods that have helped me.

Pushing through the instabilities becomes less of a struggle when we've discovered how to target specific issues within our bodies. This book is a means for me to help you take the most important steps towards nurturing your red blood cells, your organs, and your entire being in order to reap the rewards of great health you were meant to have. That's what these methods have done for me, and hopefully, you can incorporate some helpful tips and strategies to improve your situation as well.

Chapter 3
From Hopeless to Empowered: Taking Back Control

If you don't act on life, life has a habit of acting on you. You can't have all that you want if you remain the person you are. To get more from life, you need to be more in life.

– Robin Sharma

Good things come into our lives seemingly unexpectedly, though intentionally. It's no accident you and I have crossed paths for you to hear about my journey and experiences. The methods I have configured have not only improved my own health status; they have also helped other individuals and families through the process of managing and regaining health.

****

Blood Of Pain

My dis-eased body

Cannot control my eased mentality

Circulating through my veins

Is the Blood of Pain

Circulating through my veins

Is the Blood of Pain

Rage accumulates

Though sanity is maintained

My dis-eased body

Cannot control my eased mentality

****

The steps of increasing oxygen supply, building organ strength, identifying personal sensitivities in various foods and supplements, meal planning, rebuilding cells during and after an episode, and tracking my progress have been life-changing.

You no longer have to question which direction to take or what to do next. At your own pace, work through the categories and adjust step by step, or read through the

32

recommended steps once before making them part of your personal health care plan. Feel free to reach out with the contact information listed or your trusted health care practitioner for additional assistance and support. This book is designed to walk you through each process on your own.

You may already be familiar with a few of these strategies, and if so, that's great; you're ahead. If not, that's fine too. I've got you covered. If you are absolutely ready to take the steps necessary to rejuvenate yourself in natural, holistic ways, welcome. You've come to the right place.

I know it's easy to get into information overload, and not know who and what to trust. But this is our livelihood we are discussing here. We must take all information, not just with a grain of salt, but with the whole shaker!

Victory over Sickle Cell: Igniting Vibrant Health & Inspiring Transformation may just be the path that leads you to the sunny day after the storm, revealing a radiant rainbow. From proven involvement in my own health journey and through working with clients, I have no doubt that these recommendations will enhance the health of your red blood cells and entire body. This will be accomplished by strategies to increase your oxygen levels, decrease the duration and intensity of episodes, and ultimately alter your perspective on living with this fateful condition.

It's All About You

Most of us living with sickle cell anemia must learn from a young age how and why we need to adjust. Now, as a woman, I've learned that my limitations are not a hindrance, but a blessing in disguise. Yes, you did hear right. A blessing. If it wasn't for the sports I couldn't play, the trips I couldn't go on in school, the people who treated me differently, and the deep agony I've experienced over the years, my evolution towards greater health would not have happened.

Just because researchers in conventional medicine have laid out specific protocols for sickle cell patients does not mean that other methods are not valuable. It wasn't until I was finishing high school that I came to realize that I would need to be the one to get myself well.

Know thyself. These two words have tremendous implications on our health if we are careful enough to understand our unique stresses and weaknesses. Physicians, nurses, and specialists are necessary in many cases, but since you are the one living in your body and dealing with the many implications thrown your way, your desire to heal is the most important first step.

In *The Power of Your Subconscious Mind*, author Joseph Murphy writes,

If you have an intense, sincere desire to overcome a certain block in your life, if you come to a clear-cut decision that there is a way out, if you confidently decide that that is the course you wish to follow, then victory and triumph are assured.

I 100% attest to that. If you agree as well, let's begin this journey together.

The work of creating you has already been destined and manifested. Now it's about realizing that the stresses and frustrations of this condition have no place in creating our reality. They only interfere with our natural ability to help ourselves. Nurturing your physical, mental, and emotional states will collectively help you embrace the positive changes that will begin to happen. The techniques in this book will help improve communication between your conscious Self and the unconscious mechanisms of your body. This will make your wellness process much easier.

Doubts and fears are inevitable. Especially when we are going through a rough time with overall wellness, these emotions eat away at our joy for life. Yet there is a purpose for us to feel this way; it is meant to bring us towards transformation – but only if we are courageous and resilient enough to handle the pressures and circumstances that may arise.

I know you are courageous and resilient. You've had to find the strength to deal with excruciating pain from time to time (some of you in constant pain) and still have the energy to be there for your work, your family, and your home. But what about your health? If you're not well enough to take care of yourself, then what is the point of putting all your energy into everything else besides you? Hopefully, you already realize your tremendous strength as a human being. Now own it, and not just what you can do for others. This is all about you now. You matter.

Taking responsibility for your health is a lifetime job. It's only you in there, so own up to your condition – no excuses.

Strong emotions can actually bring on a crisis, something I realized as early as middle school. For every damn holiday that came up, including my birthday, I was in the hospital. Every single one! I remember getting excited for my birthday, then getting admitted. Even looking forward to a school trip. Admitted. It was awful. I had to learn how to be calm and not to exert too much energy.

Over time, holding in these emotions dragged me further down, and I lost the joy I once possessed. Can you think of an event in your life that made you realize how much this condition was interfering? There were many incidents for me, especially going through the school system, where I felt so isolated, especially in my potential.

When I participated in the triple jump in middle school, I had to be careful. When I made it to the volleyball team, there was too much pressure on my forearms. When I wanted to go into gymnastics, I was told it would be too much for my body. When I heard, "Oh, she's sickly, she can't do that," it closed my world smaller and smaller. "What the f*ck?" I thought, "Why do anything? I'll only get sick soon anyway."

That attitude stayed with me throughout school until early adulthood, when I decided that any triumph I could have over this condition was going to require my input. Being involved with medical doctors and specialists only pushed me towards taking things into my own hands. Becoming more mindful of my actions, diet, thoughts, and perspectives has had a direct impact on the length, frequency, and duration of episodes.

Acceptance is crucial for growth, allowing us to release our negative perceptions of how we deal with what we believe is beyond our control. We have no control over having sickle cell, but we have control over how we ultimately treat ourselves.

****

<u>*GET READY*</u>

Emotions radiate as one begins to dictate

Do not begin to conversate at the rate leading to hate

Don't think at a fast rate – stop

Concentrate

Consequences won't wait

When you realize it's too late

Every moment counts

Take heed of every ounce

The past reflects the present

But the present prepares for what is to come

The future – are we ready?

Gotta persevere in every situation

It takes dedication, determination

Strive for the higher power's gratification

Cut out the egotistical thought

The backbiting talks

The selfishness in walk

Or let your spirit let loose and rot

Pay attention to your surroundings

Know you can't control all things

Be aware of what radiates to others

Know we are all brotha's and sista's

Take control of your own mind and character

Let respect become your own narrator

Don't think too fast, yet don't think too slow

Let every second matter

And be prepared for yourself to grow

****

Your Navigation

You may already know your limits, or think you do, but practicing lifestyle changes in the upcoming pages will enable you to continue to push through these limitations, ultimately using them as your fuel for wellness. Everyone experiences this condition slightly differently, so there is no one way to eat or a list of supplements to take. This resource is intended to help you develop your own unique plan towards combating the negative effects of this illness. Choose the right coping mechanisms and preventative measures at your own pace for your ongoing transformative journey.

You will learn ways to assess your organ health, other than relying solely on your medical team. You will receive insight on how to increase and preserve your oxygen levels to bring health to your organs and prevent 'sickling.' You will gain an understanding of tracking your triggers as well as your progress, helping you to release mental blocks that may cause painful episodes.

Taking these practical steps on a daily basis will allow you to be a vital part of your own well-being process. Give yourself the space to concentrate on these methods and make them part of your everyday routine. Go at your own pace so this becomes a way of life. This should be something you enjoy, not just another chore that you have to do, as that would take away the satisfaction of the task at hand and your own positive energy.

Find your own personal meaning for this encounter. It is so much deeper than just physical health. It is the culmination of all those painful and frustrating times when you wished you were outside of your body so you wouldn't have to deal with such painful symptoms. The intensity and magnitude of sickle cell can be overwhelming, but allowing those feelings to overwhelm you may be doing more harm than good.

It takes time, it takes effort, but it is definitely worth it to evolve from an utter lack of hope to taking responsibility for your health. Being able to enjoy vitality and happiness is worth so much, especially when you're wishing for these states while in pain, lying on the couch, bed, or worse, in the hospital.

****

<u>*Knowing*</u>

Everything happens twice
First inside, then out
The heart and mind are powerful tools
Here's what it's all about

If sin is in your heart, then so shall you part
If deceit comes to mind, peace you will not find
If joy is omitted, dejection is permitted
If pain is penetrated, ill will is tolerated
If hate is expressed, destruction is limitless
If truth is spoken, lies are broken
If love is deep inside, life is fortified
If prayers are performed, weaknesses are transformed
If wisdom exists, various troubles are dismissed
If faith is conceived, goals are achieved
All lessons must be learned
Although some take time
Numerous virtues are earned
Life's valleys we must climb

****

If you are going through this book for the first time, you may begin by getting an overview of the following principles and methods until you understand them well enough to put them into practice. You may then go over them a second time and consider how they will fit into your personal routine and daily habits. Taking notes will help you become familiar with how your body currently functions with respect to various internal and external influences. Eventually, you'll do this with your own personalized tracking sheet. More on this in Chapter 10.

Keep this book handy to use as an ongoing reference. It is meant to guide you effectively through the most important aspect of your life: your health. Give yourself the patience and time to understand why you are putting these principles into practice and how they will benefit you, not just with managing sickle cell, but in nourishing that strong warrior you are.

Chapter 4
Oxygen Boost: Fuel Your Vitality and Thrive

Oxygen. A vital element we all need to function. Every cell in our bodies requires oxygen not only to breathe, but to survive. Have you ever felt tired, weak, short of breath, or restricted by shallow breathing? That's your body trying to conserve oxygen because it doesn't have enough to function properly.

When your cells are deprived of oxygen, it can lead to various conditions caused by ischemia (inadequate blood supply), which ultimately results in hypoxia (a deficiency in the amount of oxygen that reaches the tissues).

Here are some examples of complications that may decrease oxygen levels or interrupt blood circulation for patients with sickle cell:

Body Area	Associated Sickle Cell Complications
Brain	Stroke (lack of blood flow to the brain), Asymptomatic Cerebral Infarction (Silent Stroke)
Eyes	Retinopathy (disease of the retina), Vision Loss, Blindness
Heart	Myocardial Infarction (Heart Attack), Acute Chest Syndrome (pneumonia-like illness; leading cause of death in patients)
Muscles	Myonecrosis (localized muscle fiber death), Gangrene (death of body tissue)
Organs	Organ Damage (any), Pulmonary Hypertension (high blood pressure in the lungs), Pneumonia, Splenic Sequestration (excess sickled cells in spleen), Priapism (prolonged, painful erection)
Bone	Vaso-occlusive Bone Pain (lack of blood flow to bone), Osteonecrosis (bone death), Septic Arthritis (joint infection), Osteoporosis
Tissues	Tissue Damage, Anemia, Hand-Foot Syndrome/Dactylitis (inflamed fingers/toes), Ulcers

USING OXYGEN

Learning to enhance this vital element has made a profound difference in my life, and it absolutely can in yours. You see, the body is our temple, and when deprived of oxygen, that temple falls into crisis. In some cases, it can be fatal. But when we learn to maximize oxygen use, it can enhance our entire well-being. Every cell in our body is fueled by oxygen.

While we have had no choice but to function quite well with a lot less oxygen compared to those not afflicted with sickle cell, that doesn't give us an excuse to neglect it. We, of all people, need to optimize our oxygen levels even more by increasing supply, enhancing the function of what we already have, and maintaining balance.

Hemoglobin, the molecule within our red blood cells, carries oxygen throughout the body. In the book *Frontiers of Health,* Dr. Christine Page describes hemoglobin as carrying the "life force of joy" throughout the body. In hospitals, oxygen is, and should always be, part of the standard protocol. It is disappointing to hear otherwise in some tragic cases. Oxygen is a life force for our cells. Life force = joy for our red blood cells.

How do you feel in pain? Not joyful, that's for sure. Increasing our oxygen levels gives us a far better chance of reducing the frequency and severity of episodes we experience. So, how do we make that happen? Great question.

WATER

Let's touch on a form of oxygen that has hydrogen attached to it. No, I won't get all scientific here, but it's something we should all increase, whether we're managing an illness or not. For those of us with sickle cell, H20 is even more important. Yes, water.

How much water should you drink daily? You've probably heard the magical number of "8 cups" (2 L), but let me tell you something – that is the bare minimum. For someone managing sickle cell, drinking that amount still leaves you vulnerable to a crisis. Your true intake depends on factors such as your weight, activity level, gender, climate you live in, health conditions, age and diet, so 8 cups is the absolute minimum you should be aiming for.

Choose water that is as alkaline as possible to provide a greater platform for homeostasis (balance) in the body.

- Purchasing alkaline water at your local health food store

- Using a pH stick to test your water

- Installing an alkaline filter for your tap at home

- Trying alkaline water filter jugs (different from some well-known household replacement filter systems, which do not alter the pH value of your water).

- Using a stainless-steel canteen so that you can refill it often, rather than drinking from plastic bottles.

You can also increase hydration through foods with high water content, such as melons (not seedless), cantaloupe, pears, cucumbers, and hydroponic lettuce.

In much of the Western world, we have access to almost limitless water, yet we limit how much we actually drink. If you don't like the taste, try to focus on how much it can benefit and protect you. There are various options for adding flavor and nutritional benefits, such as using liquid chlorophyll, fresh lemon juice, or even a pinch of sea salt (preferably Himalayan or Celtic).

When we increase our water intake, we increase the chances for oxygen to flow freely through our veins and enhance the function of our organs. Your cells will love you for this.

Note: If you have kidney issues, you should collaborate with your healthcare team to develop a personalized plan for the amount of water intake that is best for your situation.

DEEP BREATHING

Louise Hay, author of *You Can Heal Your Life*, outlines the probable causes of specific conditions and provides new thought patterns to adopt. For sickle cell anemia, she states the probable cause as a belief that one is not good enough, which destroys the very joy of life. The new thought pattern she suggests is:

"This child lives and breathes the joy of life and is nourished by love. God works miracles every day."

"Lives and breathes the joy of life" – let's focus on that, because breathing is one of the most important ways to increase your oxygen levels. How do you breathe? Is it shallow from your chest, or deep from your diaphragm? Chances are that your deep breathing, if it happens at all, is much less frequent than your shallow breathing.

Here is a simple breathing exercise:

Sit down with your feet flat on the floor if in a chair, or cross your legs if on the floor. Straighten your back and sit tall. Pull your shoulders superiorly (upward), posteriorly (back), then inferiorly (down). This is a great way to straighten your posture. Keep your shoulders and arms relaxed.

As you sit and breathe, notice how you are inhaling and exhaling. Place your hand on your abdomen. As you breathe in, do you notice your abdomen protruding outward? Do you notice your chest rising? During a proper inhale, your abdomen shouldn't be sucked in; it should protrude outward. This means you are breathing shallow from your chest rather than your abdomen. Your ribs should expand as air fills your abdomen, and then your chest should fill and rise. Once you have a full breath, reversing the process is essential. Exhale to breathe out from your chest, ribcage, then abdomen.

Slowly inhale through your nose while counting to three. Then exhale gently, letting the air release through your mouth. This should not be forced; it should be a steady breath outward. Continue practicing this exercise for 5-10 complete breaths, making sure each breath is slow, steady, and controlled.

Begin with a count of three for each inhalation and exhalation, then increase the number by one for each session. For example, in your first session, count to three. In your second session, inhale to a count of four and exhale to a count of four. Then, when comfortable with that, increase the count in your next sessions to five, then six, then seven, and so on, up to 10. This exercise can be practiced multiple times per day. Simply being mindful of how you're breathing can definitely improve your overall health.

James Nestor, author of *Breath: The New Science of a Lost Art*, writes:

"It turns out that breathing at a normal rate, our lungs will absorb only about a quarter of the available oxygen in

the air. The majority of that oxygen is exhaled back out. By taking longer breaths, we allow our lungs to soak up more in fewer breaths."

It is important not to hold your breath under any circumstances. Sickled cells are highly affected by a lack of oxygen. While some deep breathing techniques require frequent holding of the breath at the peak of inhalation and exhalation, holding your breath with oxygen-deprived cells has the possibility of doing more harm, in my opinion. A continuous breathing flow without pauses encourages less stagnation. Find a breathing exercise or breathwork facilitator in your area for additional guidance if needed.

Do you find yourself breathing through the mouth? Research suggests this can also actually do more harm than good. Mouth-breathing should be avoided whenever possible, with exceptions such as during exercise or when having a bowel movement. There are numerous studies indicating that breathing this way creates more dysfunction in the body, including physical and mental stress. Did you know that mouth-breathing also contributes to periodontal disease, bad breath, and is the number one cause of cavities? It also contributes to snoring and sleep apnea. Think about that for a moment. This can be backed by hundreds of dentists, including Dr. Mark Burhenne, a renowned dentist who has been studying the links between oral health and the body for decades. He highlights that breathing through the nose can boost nitric acid six-fold, which is one of the reasons we can absorb eighteen percent more oxygen this way than by just breathing through the mouth.

All in all, deep breathing creates a rhythmic three-part breath (abdomen, ribs, and chest), which allows you to develop and use your full lung capacity while oxygenating your blood and stimulating your lymphatic and circulatory systems.

EXERCISE

Controlled breathing is also an important function in exercise. Yes, intense exercise will be out of the question in most cases, but that's no excuse to not do *any*. To maximize your oxygen levels, it's important to dedicate time to getting you (and your cells) moving to improve circulation. Anything that can essentially get your heart pumping a bit faster (without overexertion) will enhance your hemoglobin levels, thereby decreasing the potential for cell clumping or clotting in a particular area.

Yoga is an exercise that not only focuses on breathing, but also on increasing the function of your body's organs and systems, improving flexibility, and connecting you with your inner self. All of this provides significant relief from sickle cell symptoms.

There are various types of yoga you can experiment with, which are extremely beneficial, and no, you don't have to go out and join a yoga studio. You can purchase a DVD or use online resources. Start with something geared towards beginners and go from there. It is important to enjoy the chosen session so that it's easier to make this activity a regular habit.

Whatever exercise routine you choose, your primary goal is to increase your oxygen supply by connecting it with the pattern of your breath, while moving through different positions to maximize your blood flow, and improve your bone health.

ENVIRONMENTAL AWARENESS

Once we're getting used to breathing more optimally and engaging in proper movement, it's time to turn our attention to the products we use within the home. Are you drinking from plastic BPA bottles? Are you using the microwave often? What products are you using to clean your home? What are you putting on your skin?

These decisions can greatly increase the amount of oxidation stress you place on your cells. To understand oxidation, think of an apple. When you slice an apple and it is exposed to the air, it will eventually start to brown. When this happens in your body, it is unable to perform essential tasks to function easily. Cells start to malfunction, get damaged, and break down. Adding lemon juice to a cut apple, which contains antioxidants, inhibits the oxidation process. Like lemon juice to a cut apple, antioxidants such as the phytochemicals found in fruits, vegetables, legumes, nuts, and seeds protect our cells against the damaging effects of oxidation.

Furthermore, the pH specifications of not only water, but also food, are important to note here. As research indicates, blood carries oxygen to your cells at an alkaline pH of approximately 7.4. If this pH slides lower than 7.4 (leading to acidosis) or above (leading to alkalosis), it will decrease energy production and the oxygen-carrying capacity of the blood.

We mostly live in an acidic environment and create acidic environments for ourselves (high stress, toxic food, negative thoughts/emotions, high-intensity activities), and so keeping our bodies less overburdened by being less acidic, limiting our exposure to unnecessary chemicals, is truly worth the effort.

HYDROTHERAPY

Hydrotherapy increases your oxygen supply by using the properties of water to effectively penetrate deep into your tissues. It is defined as using water, either externally or internally, in the treatment of trauma or disease. This water can be in the form of a solid, liquid, or vapor. Herbal and chemical preparations may also be applied, including plasters, poultices, masks, wraps, and baths.

There are a few who benefit from a localized cold application for pain relief, although most individuals with sickle cell disease benefit from heat. You see, when your body is tense, everything constricts. Imagine jumping into a pool of cold water, or even dipping your feet in cold water alone. Your body tenses up, and you start shivering. Even the thought of that can have similar effects. This is your body's way of conserving heat.

Heat is vitally important for patients with sickle cell. For one, we were not meant to be in cold climates. Our very condition solidifies that our ancestors were not from cold climates. Why force that environment on ourselves? Many of us don't have a choice in where we currently live, but that gives us more reason to look into hydrotherapy.

When in physical pain, deep, moist heat is more effective than a heating pad. Heating pads provide heat and relief, but they do not penetrate deeply into your tissues. Deep, moist heat from a hydrocollator can significantly increase your chances of that heat getting to where it needs to be, which is beneath your tissues and not just on the surface of your skin. When heat penetrates beneath your tissues, it optimizes your cells to become more free-flowing, which is what they're asking for. They're not asking for temporary relief; they need this close stimulation to move out of the "jam" they're in.

CRYOTHERAPY

As previously mentioned, a few individuals benefit from localized cold application for pain relief. Recently, cryotherapy has taken me by surprise. I have been experimenting with this therapy for a few years now, and have experienced amazing benefits.

This nitrogen-gas-based cold therapy involves up to 3 minutes of skin exposure with temperatures reaching –150 to –180°C. It can be used for a local application, a full body session, or both. Since it is totally different from cold that is moist (the outdoors, water, etc.), this dry cold from nitrogen gas is for anyone looking to restore and revive cellular activity. Regular treatments have been shown to decrease inflammation, swelling, and pain, and may also reduce the frequency and severity of episodes.

With regular use, cryotherapy can drastically promote increased oxygenation of cells, mental calmness, stress relief, joint and muscle recovery, and better sleep. If you have any form of sickle cell or are interested in overall wellness, consider learning about the many benefits of cryotherapy and trying it if you're willing.

I recommend starting with spot or localized treatments (one area or limb at a time), then progressing to full-body sessions when comfortable and mentally prepared. Start with up to one minute or a minute and a half, and then increase gradually, possibly 5-10 seconds at a time, to your own limit.

Three minutes isn't suitable for everyone. Due to the numerous personal and medical factors at play, you must err on the side of caution with anything new and drastic and give yourself enough time between sessions so that you can assess its effectiveness.

MASSAGE THERAPY

"Massage has a positive effect on all body systems. It has been recognized as effective in reducing nociceptive (painful) nerve firing. One study concluded that massage is beneficial for myofascial pain and muscle tension. Massage can break the pain cycle and eliminate the original source of the pain by increasing blood flow to the ischemic tissue." (Kisner & Colby, 1996; Juhan, 1987).

Specific techniques help to relax muscles, decrease spasms, break down adhesions, release trigger points (muscle "knots"), improve lymphatic flow, remove metabolic waste, increase respiratory capabilities and immune function, and decrease nervous system firing. Most importantly, massage reduces stress, anxiety, and depression. Since stress lowers immune response, it increases susceptibility to illness. Protecting our systems with regular massage therapy will enhance our total body wellness.

Although many forms are available, relaxation, hot stone, deep tissue (limited), Thai, trigger point therapy, lymphatic drainage, and cupping work exceptionally well for those with sickle cell. Find a good registered or licensed massage therapist to assist you with your individual needs.

As with any profession, many massage therapists are not as therapeutic as they can be, and some practitioners don't adhere to the essential principles of the practice. Before you begin working with a therapist, find out how much they know about your condition and whether they have experience treating others with sickle cell or any other issues you're dealing with. This will enhance your chances of receiving the treatment you require and deserve.

As Jethro Kloss states in the book *Back to Eden* (Revised & Updated version):

"The structures directly affected by massage are the skin with its underlying fat and connective tissue, muscles, blood vessels (both arteries and veins), lymph channels, nerves, bones, joints, and ligaments. Indirectly affected are the heart, lungs, and large organs within the abdomen. Massage is one of the most valuable remedial measures. When used in combination with water treatments, it accomplishes amazing results. It assists in building up the blood by increasing the hemoglobin and the total number of red blood cells, and it rebuilds the tissues in general."

You can attest that these benefits are profound!

If your cells are struggling to function with the limited oxygen they already have, coupled with the stresses we continue to place on our bodies, it depletes those oxygen levels even more. Breathing, taking note of environmental products, increasing water through food and drink, exercising, hydrotherapy, cryotherapy, and massage therapy all provide ways to increase your oxygen levels. This, in turn, can decrease the intensity and duration of a crisis and lengthen the duration between them.

Increasing oxygen = increasing vitality, joy, and happy cells.

Chapter 5
Power Up: Strengthen Your Organs for Resilience

Organ damage is a common occurrence with a sickle cell diagnosis, so we need to work with and not against our natural bodily functions. Having sight matters. Having independently functioning kidneys, gallbladder, and spleen matters. Having healthy, longer-lasting red blood cells matters. It is a matter of life and death.

Paying attention matters.

What if you didn't have to worry about additional doctor's visits on top of the regular appointments you should already be following up with? Wouldn't you have more time to pay attention to things that are important to you? Understanding your body's requirements takes both patience and action from you. It takes that will inside you that says, *"I need to take advantage of my health and not leave it completely in the hands of anyone else."*

Who else truly knows what you're going through except for you? Who else knows what's going on in your mind when you're going through a painful episode? Living with this condition has many limitations, but like the fighters we are, we must continue to combat them with love and care through the choices we make.

Here, we will focus on your major body organs and systems in relation to the health of your red blood cells. When your body is fighting off bacteria or viruses, it manifests as weakness, such as a cold or infection. Constipation shows up as an upset stomach, bloating, and irritability. A crisis manifests as physical pain.

Whenever we experience discomfort, that's our body's way of communicating with us. It talks to us all the time, but do we listen? Usually, we don't take action until symptoms are screaming in our faces, forcing us to submit. Why not take action before anything happens? No, we can't always guess when we're going to have an episode, but we can definitely take action to prevent them as often as possible. If we do this, then our bodies will thank us with better health and fewer attacks.

To support the internal functioning of your cells, consider paying attention to the organs and systems you may have slightly more issues with, and then work towards supporting that organ.

Here is a list of organs categorized by system:

Body System	Organs/Structures Included
Digestive	Mouth, Tongue, Esophagus, Stomach, Pancreas, Small Intestine, Liver, Gallbladder, Rectum, Anus, Mesentery
Intestinal	Colon (Large Intestine), Small Intestine, Sigmoid Colon, Rectum, Anus
Circulatory/Cardiovascular	Heart, Blood, Arteries, Veins, Capillaries
Nervous	Brain, Spine, Spinal Cord, Senses
Immune/Lymphatic	Spleen, Lymph, Lymph Nodes, Thymus, Tonsils, Adenoids, Appendix
Respiratory	Lungs, Throat, Pharynx, Larynx, Bronchioles, Alveoli, Sinus, Diaphragm
Urinary	Bladder, Kidney, Urethra, Ureters
Glandular/Endocrine	Pituitary, Pineal, Thyroid, Parathyroid, Thymus, Adrenals, Organs of Reproduction, Liver, Pancreas
Musculoskeletal	Hair, Skin, Nails, Bones, Tendons, Joints, Ligaments, Cartilage,

	Muscles, Connective Tissues
Reproductive	Vagina, Uterus, Ovaries, Fallopian Tubes, Cervix, Penis, Scrotum, Testes, Epididymis, Spermatic Cord, Ductus Deferens, Seminal Vesicles, Ejaculatory Duct, Urethra, Prostate

Sickle cell complications can arise in any of these systems. Let's take a closer look at them to better understand what imbalances may occur.

DIGESTIVE SYSTEM

The digestive system can be considered the gateway to health. This is the only place where the substances we eat and drink can be broken down and metabolized. As we learned in the previous chapter, red blood cells carry oxygen throughout the body. Whatever is granted entrance through our "food doorway" (the mouth) can affect its relationship with your cells once they encounter it. Imbalances here can affect all other body systems.

"All the rules of prudence or gifts of experience that life can accumulate will never do as much for human comfort and welfare as would be done by a stricter attention and a wiser science directed to the digestive system."

– Thomas DeQuincy (1785-1876)

INTESTINAL SYSTEM

You cannot effectively eliminate waste from your body without a properly functioning intestinal system. The colon is often referred to as the body's most important organ. Since the intestinal wall is coated with billions of microorganisms (healthy and unhealthy flora/bacteria), dietary intake must be optimal.

Aside from food, our systems have also been inundated with medication after medication. As you know, we require powerful pain medicine, and there are times when we need ample doses to relieve symptoms. Of all the side effects that may occur, this has a negative effect on the ability to eliminate what does not belong. Drugs are completely foreign, alter biochemical reactions, and deal with symptoms, not causes. Drugs are necessary when required, though the effects can cause ongoing imbalances, decreasing our resistance to illness and infections. This, in turn, can develop into a crisis simply by the system being "backed up."

Constipation is a common issue during and after a crisis, usually due to medication taken. How often do you have a bowel movement? Daily? Weekly? If your bowel movements are once or less per day, you can consider yourself constipated. Imbalances here, too, can affect all other body systems.

CIRCULATORY SYSTEM

The circulatory system enables the body to efficiently transport nutrients in and out of cells, ensuring the proper functioning of the entire structure. It is obvious when we feel a lack of circulation. In general, we feel more lethargic, and that can create more tension in the body.

For those of us diagnosed with sickle cell, when blood cannot properly flow to where it needs to be, it can easily get concentrated in specific areas such as the arms, legs, back, head, gluteal muscles, or virtually anywhere blood flows. When this happens, it creates a perfect environment for red blood cells to clump together, leading to general weakness and pain.

Imbalances in this area can affect all other body systems, particularly the nervous, respiratory, and gastrointestinal systems.

NERVOUS SYSTEM

The nervous system is one of the most critical, simply because it involves the brain and spinal cord. Nerves from the spinal cord connect to every organ in the body. As we know, strong emotions can have a major impact on how our cells react. When we are feeling a particular emotion, it sends a signal to our organs.

What are your predominant thoughts? Any strong emotion can give a big jolt of electricity to different parts of the body. This will then stimulate adrenaline, shutting down unnecessary areas (such as digestive functions) to focus on the task at hand, making it easier for cells to become concentrated in a particular area, which can lead to pain.

Imbalances here can affect all other body systems, so learning to maintain a state of serenity is important.

IMMUNE/LYMPHATIC SYSTEM

The ability to resist infections is of high concern for patients with sickle cell disease. The musculoskeletal system is associated here for the reason that the bone marrow stem cells (originating in the bone) mature to become white and red blood cells. Our white blood cells are considered soldiers of the immune system, which require specific nutrients to stimulate their production, growth, and the ability to immobilize dangerous microbes directly.

There are no resources to fight back when one's body is poorly nourished. Dr. Laila O. Afrika has noted that on a natural foods diet, sickle cell anemia does not pose a problem. A diet of processed foods, meats, dairy, drugs, white sugar, salt, etc., has the potential to destroy not only vital nutrients but also white blood cells, making you more susceptible to infection and other complications.

"The road to better health will not be found through more drugs, doctors, and hospitals. Instead, it will be discovered through better nutrition and changes in lifestyles."

– William Crook, MD

Helping to boost your body's own defense mechanisms can assist in preventing sickle cell episodes, reducing the potential for infections to arise, and decreasing the duration and recovery time of episodes.

RESPIRATORY SYSTEM

All cells need oxygen. Oxygen is life. The respiratory system supplies fresh oxygen to the blood, which can then be distributed to all body tissues. As we learned in the previous chapter, breathing from the diaphragm as opposed to shallow breathing from the chest assists the body in gathering sufficient oxygen to supply our tissues and organs.

Compromised breathing can trigger a crisis. Of all the involuntary processes conducted within our amazing machinery, breathing is both voluntary (conscious) and involuntary (unconscious).

Daily exposure to air pollution, smoking (both firsthand and secondhand), and factors affecting breathing rates can impact the optimal functioning of this system. These factors would include exercise, mood, certain medications, and stress. Imbalances here can affect the immune, circulatory, and nervous systems.

URINARY SYSTEM

Regulating the volume and composition of fluids in the body and keeping an internal chemical balance of electrolytes and metabolites are the main functions of the urinary system. Do you pay attention to your urine? Have you noticed the colors being red, brown, amber, dark yellow, yellow, light yellow, or clear? It indicates healthy or unhealthy regulation of fluids. In some cases, especially urine with a red tint, may indicate food residues – like that of eating beets.

pH balance is also regulated here. Therefore, the amount of acidity may be identified by the pH balance of your urine (or even saliva). Imbalances here can affect glandular and circulatory systems, especially the reproductive organs, adrenal glands, and major blood vessels.

GLANDULAR SYSTEM

"If you skew the endocrine system, you lose the pathways to self. When endocrine patterns change, it alters the way you think and feel. One shift in the pattern tends to trip another."

– Hilary Mantel

Regulating functions such as stress response, metabolism, growth, and sexual reproduction, the glandular system is responsible for most of our well-being. Recovering from extremely painful sickle cell episodes, surgeries, treatments, not to mention personal and social issues, it is continuously taxed, whether or not a crisis is present.

Ongoing stressful situations not only deplete our nutrition stores, but also the hormones that need to be secreted to properly regulate all biological processes in the body. These hormones are chemical messengers secreted into the bloodstream to carry out various functions via the organs, muscles, and other tissues.

Imbalances here can affect the digestive, reproductive, nervous system, and circulatory systems.

MUSCULOSKELETAL SYSTEM

The musculoskeletal system is of particular significance because the skeletal system is where bone marrow is located. It is within the bone itself where white blood cells, platelets, and most importantly, red blood cells are produced. Since our red blood cells die faster than those of other individuals (normal red blood cells live 90-120 days, whereas sickle cells last only 10-20 days), we must be able to help increase and sustain the longevity of our red blood cells through supplementation, food, and lifestyle habits.

Contrary to popular opinion, it is healthy protein and fat options, high complex carbohydrates including an abundance of fresh vegetables and fruit, whole grains, nuts and seeds, along with weight-bearing exercises that promote bone health – not in drinking milk.

Recent studies have reported that dairy has the potential to *increase* the risk of osteoporosis. Countries with the highest consumption of dairy confirm increased mortality, bone fractures, and bone loss in the same population. It has also been considered "liquid meat," as it may contain similar amounts of saturated fat and cholesterol as red meat.

Every time we have a crisis, it "eats away" at our bones. Supporting the health of our skeletal system helps to repair some damage that has already been done. Imbalances here can affect all other body systems.

REPRODUCTIVE SYSTEM

Survival of the species is the primary function of the reproductive system. It is a choice to pass on the mutated hemoglobin gene (HbS) to your offspring, so careful thought must be considered. For many of us warriors, such as myself, this choice wasn't a thought; I had learned it. My parents had no idea that they were even carriers of this mutated gene. As a result, the challenging road ahead was a tremendous experience and a journey that came with a lot of lows.

Research has shown that fertility affects both men and women who have been diagnosed with sickle cell anemia. Sperm abnormalities in males, along with risk factors that may inhibit females from conceiving, may affect the likelihood of conception. Though, as we clearly understand, many women have been able to carry out successful pregnancies despite this condition.

The health of your reproductive organs can play a large role in the functioning of your endocrine and urinary systems.

In supporting our systems, we can make it easier for our entire body to function at a better rate and achieve homeostasis, even with its limited resources.

NURTURING YOUR CELLS

High-quality whole food sources, herbs, and nutrients can significantly improve your health when you choose to support your own wholeness. What can you learn from an episode? Even if it's one of those random attacks, take this time to reflect on your stress levels, workload, and personal purpose.

Think of it as a test. A test to see how far you can go before your next episode. A test to see how beneficial nutrients can support your body to perform its necessary functions without reminding you of painful symptoms. As Les Brown puts it, *"No test, no testimony."* Aren't you here currently reading to learn how to restore your body? Let's do this.

First, pay attention to where your body needs help the most. Which of your organs and/or systems needs the most assistance? Have you been affected or diagnosed with other medical issues, such as frequent colds or infections (immune/lymphatic), diabetes (glandular, digestive), high cholesterol (circulatory/cardiovascular, digestive), asthma (respiratory), osteoporosis, and muscle or joint and bone issues (musculoskeletal), or depression (nervous, glandular)?

Can you see correlations here? What organs or systems have you had issues with? This is how you can narrow down your most compromised areas. Give additional attention to these areas by way of supplementation and foods, then experience the benefits of fewer episodes because of the nourishment you will be providing for your body. It will no longer have to ask for attention by way of adverse symptoms. When you communicate with your body by recognizing what it needs, you can live a life of enhanced vitality.

****

POISON

Species become ill by me

Mentally and physically

I am foul, POISON, and contaminate

To make the clean impure

You endure me yet despise me.

You make me, yet want to destroy me

Why am I here?

I do no good...

Terminate me from your air, your lungs

Your food, your drink

Tolerate not the harsh reality.

Put my existence to an end

Sanitize Mother Earth

And appreciate her worth

Chapter 6
Holistic Insights: Uncover Hidden Imbalances

Our microbiome (the collection of all microorganisms in and on our bodies, such as bacteria, viruses, fungi, and one-celled protozoa) plays a crucial role in maintaining balance within our internal environment. It helps us regulate our immunity, mental health, and digestive health.

Sneezing, coughing, skin eruptions (acne, rashes, etc.), and inflammation are all ways the body tries to rid itself of potentially harmful substances. Whether or not your body is speaking to you in these ways, it is constantly battling an off-balance internal environment. In today's world, we are bombarded with pollution, processed foods, and radiation from microwaves, laptops, cell phones, tech gadgets, and the overall advances of modern technology.

"If we could eliminate certain outside frequencies that interfered with our bodies, we would have greater resistance to disease."

– Nikola Tesla

We need to focus on lessening the episodes that could ultimately cause our demise. Even between episodes, when you are considerably well and not in extreme pain, you may still feel weak. You may be constantly fighting infections, taking antibiotics, or undergoing medical treatments. Your body is constantly working on effectively managing the situation.

Our sensitivity to factors in our environment is making our blood cells fight a fight they cannot win alone. Through a non-invasive process, a sensitivity evaluation can reveal the effects certain substances, such as heavy metals, supplements, and food items, may be having on your overall health. We can screen for the efficacy of nutritional supplements, the energetic presences of parasites, candida, viruses, and bacteria, and determine any nutritional deficiencies. In this way, an individualized plan can be recommended to help normalize your cell function.

FIGURING OUT INDIVIDUAL WEAKNESSES

If our red blood cells live only about 20 days instead of the usual 120, we cannot afford to keep exposing our bodies to items and situations that progressively stress and weaken our systems. Taking a proactive approach to finding out your unique sensitivities may give clues as to why you have frequent episodes or why it takes a long time to recover.

There is a saying, *"If you don't eat your food as medicine, you'll have to then eat medicine as your food."* How many medications are you currently on? How many more are added when you are enduring an episode? Pain medications alone alter the body's internal environment. Now, just imagine the total quantity of medications you've taken up to this point, then seriously consider the effect they have had on the internal balance of your microbiome.

Our organs must work harder to process and get rid of these foreign substances, which leaves us with residual damage, affecting our internal balance and hindering our health even further. When sensitivities develop and heavy metals accumulate, it becomes even more important to know exactly what your body requires to achieve and maintain vibrant health.

Yes, certain nutrients generally have positive effects, but we also know that what benefits one person may have no effect on another, or even a negative effect. Failing to recognize your unique needs can compromise the efficiency of how your cells function and hinder your progress.

MERIDIAN STRESS ASSESSMENT/BIOSCAN

One way to accurately pinpoint which systems are most compromised is through a BioScan. This is a non-invasive procedure incorporated into my practice, and I have seen first-hand impressive improvements for both myself and my clients using this method.

A BioScan is a Meridian Stress Assessment (MSA) that measures energetic organ frequencies using Electroacupuncture According to Voll (EAV). Dr. Reinhard Voll, a German medical doctor and engineer, reasoned that if acupuncture theory was correct and channels of energy (also referred to as *chi*, *prana*, *ka*, or *vital life force*) did indeed run throughout the body, there should be a way to measure this energy.

In the book *Blueprint for Immortality*, Harold Saxton Burr states that electrical properties exist wherever there is life. Modern physics also demonstrates that matter and energy are interrelated, with matter being viewed as a denser form of energy. Therefore, imbalances and diseases in the physical body are the result of disturbances in the energy field of a particular organ or system. Meridians are the pathways through which this energy or electric current flows.

EAV is a great way to discover weaknesses you may not have known otherwise. Not only does it recognize weaknesses and stresses, but it can also give you individualized recommendations for nutrients that can directly address each weakness. This helps to provide a comprehensive review of your entire body, giving a clear profile of your present condition. Each area of the body (whether it be an organ or a system) is evaluated and determines results in either a *balanced*, *stressed*, or *weakened* state.

This technique is used to measure the electrical conductance or resistance at responsive meridian points, most often located on your fingers and toes. During the assessment, you simply hold a brass rod in one hand while the MSA technician touches the tip of a brass probe on specific points on your hand or foot. The MSA device then measures the skin's resistance to the minute amount of electrical signal passing through the probes.

Picture your spine as the hub, with nerves radiating outward, connecting to and surrounding the organs and systems throughout your entire body. These nerves and meridian points extend towards your extremities on your fingers and toes. Once pressure is placed at those particular points during the assessment, a signal is sent to the corresponding area (such as the nervous system point or the cellular metabolism point). You can instantly see whether changes should be made, and in what ways. With this method, not only will you see your results right away, but a detailed report will also provide specific recommendations to enhance your most compromised areas, based on your own body's tolerance to certain whole foods and supplements. If a BioScan is not accessible, alternatively, you may download the Body System Questionnaire located in the Resources tab on our website at www.essentialhealingsolutions.ca which can also help you decipher your most compromised organs and systems.

Yes, we all need a healthy diet routine consisting of leafy greens and vegetables, healthy protein, oils, and grains, along with fruits, nuts, and seeds. But the key is figuring out how to address your unique weakest links, as it can vastly improve your potential to rebuild health. Identifying your specific areas of need will give you this advantage.

FREQUENCIES FOR LIFE/HEALY

More recently, adding frequency therapy has proven successful in optimizing my cellular function. More precise areas of the auric field, as well as mental and biological facets, can be evaluated and harmonized to their best potential. Unlike the BioScan, **Healy** is a small, wearable device designed for both personal and professional use. Compact and convenient, it helps to detect imbalances and provide the necessary frequencies to support optimal wellness. This device uses frequency therapy to stimulate specific areas of the body and helps support the restoration of the cell membrane tension to its most beneficial level.

Functioning with approximately 30 trillion cells, we've learned that our body is as healthy as the health of these cells and their ability to communicate with each other. Since our cells respond to signals in our environment, from what we touch and how we move, we must be careful and aware of what implications this may have. Tissues and organs will become compromised if our cells do not operate efficiently.

Cytologists Dr. Robert O. Becker and Dr. Bjorn Nordenstrom, former chairman of the Nobel Prize Committee, discovered that almost all acute and chronic illnesses may have been caused by a decrease in the cell's membrane voltage. By analyzing the bioenergetic field of the body in real time, it is now possible to not only determine where support is needed but also deliver the right frequencies into the body to help regenerate at the cellular level.

Frequency therapy, by way of using the Healy device, makes it that much easier to harmonize specific areas impacted by internal and external stressors. Areas evaluated are to instantly assist cells, including the energetic activation, balancing, and promoting cell health through the harmonization of your own bioenergetic field.

As a holistic practitioner, this integration just makes sense. Harmonizing your bioenergetic field cannot be done through physical aspects like food and drink alone. In the current world we live in, there are multiple insults externally in our environment, which in turn affect us internally.

Having access to a device such as the Healy has dramatically impacted the functioning of my cells.

HAIR MINERAL ANALYSIS

"All chronic and degenerative diseases are caused by two and only two major problems: TOXICITY and DEFICIENCY."

— Charlotte Gerson.

Learning about your body's state of deficiencies and excesses can catapult you in the right direction toward improved health. Hair, as a soft tissue, offers a permanent record of the body's nutritional status, making it an ideal material for assessing mineral balance.

Hair is a body tissue that passes through the lymph, blood, and extracellular fluids before reaching the skin's surface. As the outer layers harden, the metabolic products gathered during their formation become permanently locked in.

Minerals are crucial for nearly all enzyme reactions, metabolic processes, and detoxification in the body. Even in small amounts, they are essential for absorbing and utilizing nutrients effectively.

Unlike blood tests, which only show what's circulating at a specific moment, hair provides a three-month snapshot of mineral levels and toxic elements stored within your cells.

When I completed my first Hair Mineral Analysis, the results were as enlightening as they were alarming. Elevated levels of heavy metals like aluminum and lead were wreaking havoc on my system. At the same time, essential minerals such as magnesium and zinc, critical for energy and immunity, were severely depleted. This wasn't just data; it was a reflection of how my body had been silently screaming for help.

The report was eye-opening. It revealed why my energy had been so erratic, why my mind sometimes felt foggy, and even why my emotions had been like a rollercoaster. The relationship between minerals and health is intricate, like a symphony; one imbalance can throw the entire orchestra out of tune. But what stood out the most was the realization that no "one-size-fits-all" diet or supplement regimen could address these deeply personal imbalances.

Through the tailored recommendations from my hair analysis, I began replenishing what I lacked while assisting in the removal of harmful elements stored in my tissues. The changes were slow but steady. My energy started to stabilize, my mind became clearer, and my mood evened out. What once felt like insurmountable challenges suddenly became manageable.

ENERGETIC AWARENESS

"Don't think there are no crocodiles just because the water is calm."

– Malawian proverb

While the Hair Mineral Analysis addressed biochemical needs, energetic assessments helped me understand how unresolved stress and suppressed emotions were quietly draining my vitality. By working on both the physical and energetic levels, I reached a level of healing that felt truly holistic.

During those rare times when you experience little to no pain, do you tend to overdo it? I've surely had my moments, which only left my body stressed and drained. Instead, let's use those times of wellness to extend their duration and prolong that joy and health. Identifying your major weaknesses gives you a better understanding of how you may want to treat your body.

How our different organ systems function correlates energetically (as practiced with Reiki & the Chakras) with our foundation, relationships, will, self-love, communication, intuition, and purpose in life. Holistic health is not only about your physical symptoms; it involves your whole being. This is why choosing to incorporate a holistic approach when communicating with and assisting our bodies is imperative.

DO NOT IGNORE YOUR SYMPTOMS

Back in 2018, I was working pretty much seven days a week for up to 12 hours each day. At this time, I was a full-time massage therapist working with multiple companies and also providing in-home services. My body was easily able to capture a virus. My time of the month was right around the corner (which usually increases my chances of having a mild-severe episode), and I was neglecting my health in terms of sleep. All these factors, combined with some personal and planetary matters (sensitive to moon cycles and energies), conspired to completely shut down my body.

I started to get aches, developed cold symptoms, and was beyond exhausted, but I still kept pushing through. As much as we sickle cell warriors try to endure our pain, beware. You will only do yourself more harm. The pain escalated and was so severe that I ended up in the hospital. I had to be escorted by ambulance from my bedroom. I remember the paramedics were reluctant to provide enough pain medication on the way to the hospital because they were shocked at what I was already taking to try to manage the pain on my own. It obviously had no effect. No one should ever have to experience what we do.

This is why we need to pay attention to the very source of our health: by listening to our body, understanding our limitations, and taking the necessary steps to get well and stay that way for as long as we can. Our immune system may not be as strong as some, and therefore, discovering what may be lurking within our cells to enhance our well-being doesn't seem so far-fetched.

I was released from the hospital after about six days, but was still very weak. When I had the energy to complete a BioScan food and organ assessment of my own, my eyes widened in disbelief. The results indicated there may be a potential pathology on the way, and that I was in a cellular degeneration phase. Every single organ and system was weakened.

The evaluation process gave me a set of recommendations based on my results. My weight, metabolic age, body fat, and water percentages were also taken into consideration. After taking these personalized assessments, another potential health crisis began to reverse. Building the organs and systems in most dire need of support enabled my body to restore itself, allowing those weakened areas to progress, showing balanced points that weren't present before.

You may think you know what to eat; you may have researched which foods are beneficial for sickle cell, but what if one of those items has the potential to aggravate your unique internal environment for the worse instead of for the better?

Fatigue, depression, anger, sadness, and irritability are already something we are familiar with. Still, there is always something underlying how we're feeling and functioning because of what's really going on within the cells. You may be getting over the effects of a virus, bacteria, heavy metals, or a parasite. Convalescence can be difficult, and this steals time from our joy. What if you could be proactive in your own wellness? What changes would you make to your nutrition, mindset, and/or activity levels in response to the symptoms you were being bombarded with?

NOT LEAVING IT TO CHANCE

Things probably won't work themselves out to our liking if we just let them happen. With today's technology, our will, and some proactivity, we can accomplish things we never knew were possible until we put in the effort.

It's great to get into the habit of prioritizing yourself. Take the current knowledge you have, implement the necessary steps, then continuously improve on that. Discovering potentially harmful substances within your body not only gives you tools to better communicate with your amazing machinery, but also provides great insight into how to negate the harmful effects of adverse substances.

My clients notice substantial improvement in undesirable symptoms when they alter their food choices and incorporate small steps to improve their current state of health. Start with the basics: Enhance your diet with real, live, whole foods; continuously enhance your oxygen supply; and truly listen to your body. Then narrow down what you may be sensitive to, what underlying causes may be affecting you genetically, and the stresses and weaknesses that may be reducing your potential to heal more effectively.

We must acknowledge and understand that the dimensions of the physical world we live in could not exist without the initial energetic frequencies that enable all to currently manifest. Paying attention to the nutrients ingested daily is essential. Tapping into the deeper aspects of our existence does not stop here. Energy therapy is nothing new. Considering the onslaught of multiple attacks on the vitality of our cells and organs, frequency therapy is one of the best ways to accelerate your individualized vibrancy.

In my personal and professional experience, getting a comprehensive profile of your physical and energetic condition reveals valuable insights and accurate methods for recognizing and removing blockages that you may not have otherwise been aware of.

Just as we shouldn't leave life to chance, this also applies to our health. We may have to make regular adjustments to our daily routine to accommodate the temple we've been provided with, but we also have more reasons not to leave our health to chance.

Chapter 7
Nourish Wisely: Design Your Personal Meal Plan

We all know some foods are more nutrient-dense than others, and others that are not foods at all! Now that your assessment has identified the most beneficial foods to consume, and nutrition information has been provided, a personalized plan can be devised. If you do not currently have access to these phenomenal evaluations, then start by reducing all foods high in sugar, refined carbohydrates, and saturated fats. These cause aggravations and/or sluggishness within cell walls, making the body even less efficient overall than it already is.

You want to support, not impede, the way your cells function. Supplying your body with the necessary nutrients for blood, digestion, and immunity is key. Yes, every single organ system in your body is important, but paying attention to these three areas can vastly change the way you feel and ultimately think about food. Get into the habit of fueling yourself not just because you're hungry, but because your cells need essential nutrients.

Remember the lifespan of our red blood cells? If they die off so much faster, how do you think that will impact everything else? Hemoglobin carries oxygen from the lungs to all parts of the body. A lack of oxygen anywhere can have damaging and even lethal effects. We can build on the practices from *Chapter 4* by allowing our bodies to receive oxygen from what we eat. You can start by adding more foods with high water content, such as watermelons (with seeds), cucumbers (with seeds), pears, and hydroponic lettuce.

Additionally, increase your intake of alkaline foods, such as avocados, apples, soursop, and mangoes, which help the body automatically activate its healing mechanisms. Remember our discussion of toxins in the environment and how that affects our oxygen supply? Fight this with antioxidants found in fresh berries, pomegranates, cherries, grapefruit, and dark vegetables of all colors.

CLEARING OUT THE CLUTTER

Once you know about the power of foods that help or harm you and your family, you are obligated to do something about it.

"Knowing is not enough; we must apply. Willing is not enough; we must do."

– Johann Wolfgang von Goethe

It's easy to read something and think you might just try it out. It takes commitment to continue working on yourself, not just in that moment, but for the long term. Our genetics will not suddenly change overnight.

"Genes are not just inherited; they can also be influenced by the choices we make."

– *The Gene: An Intimate History* by Siddhartha Mukherjee

First, review your kitchen – where healing can occur and diseases may start (your body becomes unhealthy long before a disease is diagnosed). What do you keep in your fridge, freezer, cupboards, and pantry? How many "non-food" items can you count? In *Drugs Masquerading as Foods*, author Suzar (Dr. S. Epps) names the five fatal foremost traits of what she calls America's killer drug foods:

1. Perverted before birth.

2. Grown in poison.

3. Sprayed with death.

4. DEAD – especially from cooking and irradiation.

5. Processed and embalmed with chemical poisons.

Non-foods are genetically modified, grown in soil deprived of nutrients by fertilizers, pesticides, herbicides, etc., and mixed with chemicals and toxic substances into a formula that tastes like food. However, your body does not recognize it as food. Eating it forces your body to use the energy it needs to continuously eliminate all these foreign substances. Please get into the habit of buying from local farmers whenever possible, and reading labels.

What are you feeding your body, your temple? And what are you feeding your children's bodies? Are they ingredients you can't even pronounce? You want to get well, but why would you start eating right and still provide your children with poison? Does that make sense? Most eating habits develop at home from a young age. You may say they'll only eat macaroni, hot dogs, or burgers. You may have been the same way as a child. But now that you are older, YOU make the rules.

If those burgers, noodles, cookies, chips, sodas, chocolates, and pastries had a danger sticker placed right front and center, would you still purchase them? Well, their danger warning is hidden in plain sight with those outrageously long scientific words. Who do these food-labelers think we are? Chemists?

If you really think about it, it's crazy that we willingly pay money for poison that's been mixed with taste-enhancing ingredients and stimulates the brain like a drug. Eating food as medicine is not as common as it used to be, but eating drugs as food has become much too common these days.

Taking drugs for our condition may be necessary when the time calls for it, as our bodies are constantly cleaning themselves of them. So why add more drugs by way of our food supply? The more hospitalizations and medications we face over the years, the more it calls for a stricter food regimen.

WHOLE, LIVE, GOOD QUALITY FOODS

Using whole, natural foods as much as possible is almost guaranteed to give you positive results, especially with your energy levels. Much of your food should consist of just one ingredient and no label at all – such as fruits, vegetables, nuts, seeds, and grains.

One whole food to consider is hemp. It is a profound healer. Hemp seeds and oil do wonders to oxygenate the blood. Hemp's excellent health benefits include being:

- A source of all essential amino acids

- High in omega-3

- Rich in antioxidants

- A source of dietary fiber

Use hemp butter, powder, flour, or seeds in your salads, yogurt, smoothies, shakes, pancakes, etc. Hemp has a rich spectrum of nutrients, including a high chlorophyll content, which helps to cleanse and restore tissues and cells and will ultimately help to restore balance if ingested in high quantities.

If you do not have access to a practitioner who works with BioScan to identify foods that may weaken or stress your system individually, consider these recommendations for foods that are more beneficial when eaten together. This is known as food combining.

Basic food combining strategy:

- Eat fruit alone (either ½ hour before a meal, or two hours after).

- Eat vegetables with grains, seeds, nuts, and legumes.

- Eat all vegetables together (starchy and non-starchy vegetables).

- Eat protein with non-starchy vegetables.

Starchy vegetables and legumes	Non-starchy vegetables and legumes
Black beans	Asparagus
Butternut squash	Bell peppers
Cassava (Yucca)	Broccoli
Chickpeas	Brussels sprouts
Corn	Cabbage
Green beans	Cauliflower
Kidney beans	Celery

Lentils	Cucumbers
Lima beans	Eggplant
Navy beans	Green beans
Peas	Kale
Pinto beans	Leeks
Plantains	Lettuce
Potatoes	Mushrooms
Pumpkin	Onions
Sweet potatoes	Radishes
Water chestnuts	Spinach
Yams	Tomatoes
	Zucchini

Vegan Protein Sources	
Food items of each category can be combined in various ways to ensure a well-rounded intake of essential amino acids and other nutrients.	
Legumes	Black beans, Chickpeas, Fava beans, Green peas (including split peas), Kidney beans, Lentils, Mung beans, Navy beans, Pinto beans
Nuts & Seeds	Almonds, Brazil nuts, Cashews, Chia seeds, Flaxseeds, Hemp seeds, Hazelnuts, Pine nuts, Pistachios, Pumpkin seeds,

	Sunflower seeds, Walnuts
Nut & Seed Butters	Almond butter, Cashew butter, Peanut butter, Sunflower seed butter, Tahini (sesame seed butter), any butter from the Nuts & Seeds category
Grains	Amaranth, Barley, Bulgur, Farro, Oats, Quinoa, Teff, Wild rice
Soy Products (Non-GMO)	Edamame, Soy milk, Soy yogurt, Tempeh, Tofu
Other Plant-Based Protein Sources	Hemp protein powder, Nutritional yeast, Pea protein powder, Seitan (wheat gluten), Spirulina
Vegetables (higher in protein)	Artichokes, Asparagus, Avocados, Broccoli, Brussels sprouts, Kale, Mushrooms, Potatoes (Russet or Yukon gold with skin), Spinach
Legume-Based Products	Bean-based pasta, Falafel (made from chickpeas or fava beans), Hummus (made from chickpeas), Lentil burgers
Sprouts	Adzuki bean sprouts, Alfalfa sprouts, Chickpea sprouts, Ezekiel bread

	(made from sprouted whole grains), Kidney bean sprouts, Lentil sprouts, Mung bean sprouts, Pea sprouts, Soy bean sprouts

- Avoid dairy.

- Avoid sweetened desserts.

- Avoid eating very large meals.

- Stop eating when you are no longer hungry, not when you are full.

- Drink sparingly with meals (no large gulps when eating, as food will be pushed through the digestive tract without effective assimilation).

Remember: whole, **live**, and of **good quality**, as nature intended it to be.

Please note: Certain nutrients in foods may interact with specific medications. You may be able to consume some of the listed foods in moderation, depending on your medication dosage and individual tolerance. It is advisable to discuss this with your doctor.

Medications & Effects on Ingestible Items		
Medication	**Ingestible Item**	**Effect**
Statins (help to lower cholesterol and prevent heart issues) Calcium channel blockers (help to lower blood pressure) Blood thinners Immunosuppressants	Grapefruit	May increase the concentration of the statin
Anticoagulants	Foods high in vitamin K: green leafy vegetables, broccoli, cauliflower	Can minimize effectiveness
Antibiotics	Dairy	Can minimize effectiveness
Alcohol	Any medication	May be dangerous and life-threatening
Caffeine	Dietary supplements Blood pressure medication Heart medication Stimulants Immunosuppressants	Can change the acidity level of the stomach, lowering absorption. Has the potential to raise blood pressure temporarily

Some antidepressants & medications used to treat Parkinson's disease	Cheese	May cause headaches and high blood pressure

****

MOTHER-FATHER SOURCE

Mother-Father source of the divine

Manifesting itself as a bright shine

A crime

To look upon it as physical, mythical

It's beyond biblical, rhythmical

Changing the seasons for life-giving reasons

Like the seeds you sow

Making morals, virtues, opportunity

And positivity grow

Sparking a light – right?

Now open your mind, unwind, and try to find

The truth that has been left behind

The justified force of that Mother-Father source

A time predictor

Spirit up-lifter

Natural law generator and #1 factor of action

In making things happen

I am

The flesh and soul of the living sun

It planted seeds, energized, and metamorphosized

Pulling me from the root to become a tree

So independent and free like the air we breathe

See?

Working hand and hand with the elements

Equals superior function and development

Giving healing powers to

Herbs and flowers and

Having that sweet-smelling aroma

To enlighten my crown

Being blessed with the silence of sound

Here, wisdom is found

No physical manifestation has my concentration

It's simply the spiritual lessons

And cosmic awareness

That filters through my blood

All from one life-giving force

Mother-Father source of the divine

Manifesting itself as a bright shine

A crime

To look upon it as physical, mythical

It's beyond biblical, rhythmical

Changing the seasons for life-giving reasons

Like the seeds you sow

Making morals, virtues, opportunity

And positivity grow

Sparking a light – right?

It's the fuel that fed my ancestors

And every single species on this earth

There's nothin' better than

The sun rising at dawn,

And in spring, feeling the warmth of its rays

And every new beginning it brings

Hearing the birds sing, each with a different ring

Blooming branches from a firm stance

Stretching forth its hands

Revealing the beauty of its command

Butterflies in the crisp air

Flying with freedom

In this massive kingdom

Greeting the spirits from none other than

The fire in the sky...

A source you cannot deny

Giving us the strength so sharp and precise

Allowing us to inhale, exhale, and grow

And providing us with the wisdom to know

The magical essence of the Universe

Earth, Stars, and Moon

Feel the galactical powers of this room

Penetration on meditation and consume

Your deep inner soul vibration

All connected to...

Mother-Father source of the divine

Manifesting itself as a bright shine

A crime

To look upon it as physical, mythical

It's beyond biblical, rhythmical

Changing the seasons for life-giving reasons

Like the seeds you sow

Making morals, virtues, opportunity,

And positivity grow

Sparking a light

Right?

****

NUTRITION FOR YOUR BODY'S SYSTEMS

Below is a list of methods, nutrients, and foods that are beneficial for sickle cell anemia, corresponding to each system. In the next section, additional items by food categories will be discussed.

The items below are condensed to give you an idea of what specific activities, supplements, foods, and herbs are essential to help direct the system toward a more alkaline blood pH level, while also removing excess mucus. Although these foods and strategies may overlap in benefits throughout other systems, they are categorized as appropriately as possible. It may take trial and error to determine the best individual treatments and recommendations for you. Collaborate with your health care provider to enhance your approach.

Digestive

Apples, avocado oil, bananas (smallest or burro kind), callaloo, cayenne pepper, cascara sagrada, coconut, cucumbers, dates, fennel, fermented L-glutamine, figs, food-combining strategies, full-spectrum enzyme supplement, ginger, limes (key limes preferred, with seeds), mangoes, papayas, prunes, quassia, sea moss, tarragon, uncooked coconut oil, uncooked olive oil, yellow dock, zucchinis.

Intestinal

Adequate water intake, avocados, bananas (burro), cascara sagrada, dates, fiber supplement (may have a constipating effect if water consumption is already low), figs, garbanzo beans, kefir, kimchi, mangoes, mushrooms, okra, prickly pear, sauerkraut.

Circulatory/Cardiovascular

Basil, blackberries, blessed thistle, cayenne pepper, chlorophyll, cucumber, folate, lily of the valley, nettle, pear, prickly pear, raspberry, red clover, regular moderate exercise, seeded grapes, squash, ubiquinol, watercress.

Nervous

Avocado oil, vitamin B12, B-complex, blessed thistle, blue vervain, Brazil nuts, chamomile, coconut oil (not heated), damiana, DHA, fonio, hemp seed oil (do not heat), hops, kale, kamut, lavender, lettuce (not iceberg), olives, omega-3, quinoa, regular meditation (reflection, action steps, manifestation), rye, sage, sea vegetables, spelt, walnuts, wild rice.

Immune/Lymphatic

Arugula, basil, bell peppers, black seed oil, blueberries, burdock, chaparral, currants, dancing, dill, elderberry, eyebright, grapeseed oil, guinea hen weed, hemp seed oil, hydrangea, kale, key limes, listening to your favorite music, lymphatic drainage massage, and specific lymphatic movement exercises, melons, mushrooms, nettle, oregano, oranges, peaches, pears, plums, quassia, red clover, rhubarb root, sarsaparilla, sea moss/Irish moss, sesame seeds, singing, soursop, tomatoes (plum & cherry), vitamin C with bioflavonoids, turmeric, white willow bark, watercress, yellow dock.

Respiratory

Bay leaf, black seed oil, blue vervain, deep-breathing techniques, elderberry, mullein, onions, sea moss, thyme.

Urinary

Cherries, hydrangea root, kegel exercises.

Glandular/Endocrine

Awareness strategies such as journaling and visualizing, Ashwagandha, blessed thistle, bladderwrack, blue vervain, burdock, CBD oil, damiana, dandelion greens, fonio, kamut, okra, prickly pear, quinoa, rye, sage, sea vegetables, spelt, stress-management techniques, valerian, wild rice, yellow dock.

Musculoskeletal

Arnica, arugula, burdock root, calcium, chickpeas, clove, collard greens, dandelion greens, elimination of dairy (may reduce overall calcium levels), hazelnuts, lavender, nettle, red clover, sarsaparilla, spirulina.

Reproductive

Damiana, hip exercises, hops, red raspberry herb, sage, valerian, yohimbe.

FOOD HABITS

Chew your food–*really* chew it. This allows nutrients to be released from the cell walls. Food is meant to be as liquid as possible before being transported to the inner walls of the intestines for absorption. Otherwise, your body will need to work even harder to complete the work that was not finished in the mouth. Our bodies already have enough to handle; we need to support the vessel we live in.

Knowing which parts of your body need support, using alkaline foods and herbs listed above in the body system categories, and choosing foods and herbs that hold a higher water content and help oxygenate the body will all make your cells happy. Once your cells are happy, you will be happy. Happy cells = happy being. So, do some kitchen cleansing. Learn about and eat the foods that will give you the most benefit and develop healthy habits.

For example, try to always bring water and food with you whenever you're out of the house. Eat before you travel, or snack on something during your commute, to make sure you're supplying your cells with the proper nutrients. Above all, try your best not to get caught in a situation where you're forced to purchase something "on the road," because this usually means fast, fake, fried, and filled with substances you don't want your body to endure. Yes, *endure*.

You may satisfy your hunger for that moment, but your cells must endure the attack of items that are neither welcomed nor recognized as nutrients long after you satisfy your hunger. Instead of happily digesting, absorbing, and metabolizing, your body now has to figure out how quickly it can rid itself of foreign material.

PLAN AHEAD

Figure out what your usual habits are in terms of hunger and food, so you can incorporate these into a new regimen that will be easier for you to follow.

Take Shauna, for example, the mom we met in *Chapter 1*. At the beginning of her busy workday, she would leave in a rush, letting the day unfold as fate dictated, and grab whatever food her senses craved at that moment. This left her with low energy, and she and her daughters were not receiving the necessary nutrients. Scheduling and making meals ahead made a profound difference to Shauna's health and the health of her family.

Once you get into this habit, it takes very little extra time to make a larger meal or multiple meals at once. These planned leftovers mean less time spent thinking about what you're going to eat the next day, or even the day after that, leaving fewer hours in the kitchen.

Think of the kitchen as your own personal healing laboratory, where you will mix and create masterpieces that your body will reward you for consuming.

When planning your meals, consider incorporating these essential food items into your daily routine.

__Note:__ The following foods have been researched and studied for their beneficial effects on the human body. This is in no way a definitive list. Balance is key in all endeavors.

Benefits include:

- Positive influence on the microbiome (prebiotic and probiotic qualities)

- Antioxidant protection

- Increasing DNA repair

- Telomere lengthening

- Improved blood flow

- Lowered inflammation

- Cell regeneration

- Immune system protection

Category	Examples
Green Leafy Vegetables	Arugula, Collard Greens, Dandelion Greens, Kale, Lettuce, Mustard Greens, Purslane, Radicchio, Sea Vegetables, Spinach, Swiss Chard, Turnip Greens, Watercress
Nuts and Seeds (incl. Butters)	Almonds, Brazil Nuts, Cashews, Chia Seeds, Coconut, Flaxseeds, Hazelnuts, Hemp Seeds, Macadamia Nuts, Pecans, Pine Nuts, Pistachios, Pumpkin Seeds, Sunflower Seeds, Sesame Seeds, Walnuts
Grains	Amaranth, Barley, Fonio, Kamut, Millet, Quinoa, Rye, Sourdough Bread, Spelt, Whole Grains, Wild Rice
Vegetables	Arugula, Asparagus, Bamboo Shoots, Bok Choy, Broccoli, Cabbage, Carrots, Cauliflower, Celery, Collard Greens, Eggplant, Endive, Green Beans, Lion's Mane Mushroom, Shiitake Mushrooms, Nopales, Okra, Olives, Onions, Peppers, Purple Potatoes, Purslane, Rutabaga, Sauerkraut, Squash, Tomatillo, Tomato (Plum and Cherry), Turnip, Zucchini
Fruits	Apples, Apricots, Black Raspberries, Blackberries,

	Blueberries, Cherries, Cranberries, Goji Berries, Grapes (Seeded), Guava, Kiwi, Limes, Lychee, Mangoes, Melons (Seeded), Nectarines, Orange, Papayas, Peaches, Pears, Pink Grapefruit, Plums, Pomegranates, Prickly Pears, Soursop, Watermelon
Legumes	Black Beans, Chickpeas, Lentils, Lima Beans, Navy Beans, Peas
Herbs, Spices & Seasonings	Basil, Bay Leaf, Black Cumin Seed, Black Tea, Burdock, Cayenne, Chili Pepper, Cinnamon, Dill, Fennel, Ginseng, Ginger, Green Tea, Guinea Hen Weed, Irish Moss, Licorice Root, Moringa, Mullein, Nettle, Oregano, Pau D'arco/Taheebo, Raspberry, Rosemary, Sage, Thyme, Turmeric, Watercress, Yellow Dock
Fermented Items	Kimchi, Sauerkraut, Sourdough Bread, Yogurt

WHEN SHOULD YOU EAT?

There are many common theories about eating according to the time of day, the season, and even when not to eat. The truth is that we all feel hungry at different times. Our lifestyle usually determines the timing. This may be influenced by when we ate last, when we woke up, or the different timings of our work and/or family schedules.

Find the routine that works for you. If you need to be up and out early in the morning, plan and prepare so you have healthy foods to take with you. Along with your meals, carry at least 2 liters of water and snacks like sliced fruits and vegetables, nuts, granola, or a protein smoothie.

A note about protein or nutrition bars and other snacks:

Don't be deceived by the many products that claim to be healthy. Check the label and decide for yourself. Look for the ones with the lowest number of ingredients, minimal non-food items, and low sugar, cholesterol, and sodium.

There's no excuse for eating poorly. Studies have shown that one in five deaths globally occur due to poor nutrition. Current research is investigating the best nutritional interventions to manage SCA. In the meantime, by working with your healthcare practitioner and applying the recommendations you've been given here, you have the potential to decrease many symptoms. Take charge, and your cells will reap the benefits.

Eating well can also help protect you against developing other conditions in addition to sickle cell disease, as well as reduce complications. Since we're constantly trying to replenish red blood cells and oxygen, it's essential to eliminate substances that can have an adverse effect, such as consuming foods that your body struggles to metabolize.

Identify your most compromised systems and eat the foods that support those systems and organs. Targeted assessments can help you do this. Know what you are sensitive to, and use your food as medicine. Always pair this support with proper digestive care.

CHANGE IS GOOD

"Growth is painful, change is painful, but nothing is as painful as staying the same."

– Dr. Sebi

Some things you may expect when changing your diet include cravings, hunger, irritability, resistance, as well as changes to bowel movements and energy levels. Remembering why these changes are essential for your wellness will make it much easier for you to make the adjustments.

The definition of insanity is doing the same thing over and over while expecting a different result. Getting a different result takes persistence and commitment if you actually want it to come to fruition. You haven't reached this point in time by doing everything right. We are constantly learning and growing. Therefore, your way of life must be adjusted. This is a way of life, not a temporary diet.

After all, we do not have sickle cell "for some time." For many, it is lifelong. Thankfully, some individuals have been able to overcome this condition through advancements in treatment, including stem cell and bone marrow transplants, as well as gene therapy. But for many of us, this is not an option.

Addressing nutrients, food sensitivities, foreign substances, and listening to your body when it speaks through symptoms (including pain) can make a profound difference in the way your body functions, and ultimately, your life.

Chapter 8
Mind Over Matter: Building Unshakeable Mental Power

"Your subconscious never sleeps. It is always on the job. It controls all your vital functions."

– Joseph Murphy, PhD, D.D
(The Power of your Subconscious Mind)

Your mental power is a critical component in dealing with the waves of emotions we experience throughout all stages of our lives, and in how we perceive ourselves. Being unwell is an entirely different experience at different stages of life, including our teenage years and adulthood.

Seeing your body change as the years progress may open a doorway to new awakening. How does your body behave now? What treatments do you need to maintain on a daily, weekly, monthly, or yearly basis? Have you noticed any changes in the frequency of episodes? All these answers can directly affect the way we think about ourselves and what our body expects of us.

Remember Shauna? When we met, she had been working as a customer service representative for five years. Her employer was understanding about her calling in sick or taking time off because of pain. She was thankful, though she felt somewhat sorry for herself for having to limit her time and finances whenever her body told her to. While her daughters had witnessed the unpredictable nature of her pain and tried to be supportive and helpful, Shauna felt down and became depressed, as she felt incapable and helpless.

You may have had similar negative thoughts about your own situation, or perhaps in the past. I know I have. The important thing here is not to linger, repeat, or think about these statements, because this only works as a detriment to your health.

Whatever you manifest first begins as a thought. Our mindset directly affects the energetic state of our cells, which, for those of us with sickle cell, has a significant impact on how we feel and how our bodies function. That's why this step should not be overlooked. When you have negative thought patterns related to anything, especially your health, it will directly impact what you intend to achieve.

Be careful about what you say, which thoughts penetrate your mind, and your overall state of mind. We are not only physical bodies, but also energetic beings that need guidance. Working constantly on doubtful and negative thinking patterns will profoundly change the way you feel and function, ultimately helping you find the joy you may have once thought would never appear.

With this being said, what are you really focusing on? What is the image, word, or feeling state you hold? How does this make you feel? Does it drag you further into despair? Or does it allow you to embrace your life lessons to be the best you can be? This is not rocket science. Unhealthy minds create unhealthy bodies. Focusing on what you truly want, rather than what you don't want, is your goal. Bring it all into motion through this action step.

"I don't want to get sick. I'm too tired for that. I'm in pain..." Although these may all be true, they call on your subconscious mind to stay in or increase that state of being. Instead, it would be helpful to change these statements to: *"I am healthy. My energy is increasing. I'm strong."* See the difference? One way states the obvious negatively, while the other allows you to shift the energetic frequency of your cells. They then have the potential to shift our entire vibration.

****

THESE DAYS

Tangled sanity

In the midst of discovery

Poisoned mind frames

Poisoned hearts, souls

Streets of fantasy

Lack of reality

Pushin' the limits of what was givin'

What She – Nature, The Creator

Has planned and forwarded

To you, I, us

Taken for granted

What have we planted?

Youth today in the sight of disarray,

Confusion, chaos, mess...

More or less, this whole globe is in distress

Thanks to vanity, war

Lies, hear the cries of the poor and money-hungry

People, people – the end is today

The end is tomorrow

Livin' in joy and livin' in sorrow

These days

These days, more matters than what is realized

Little things, precious things

Things that you cannot see

Birds, they're free

But are we?

Emancipated though contaminated, agitated

We are not amalgamated

First in line doing crime

Elemental forces

Forces doing harm beyond our control

Proving the limits

Megabytes have reached the heights

Despite the parasites that ignite like dynamite

Might this be destiny?

To what degree do we acknowledge

Circumstance, condition, certainty, actuality

Cruelness, happiness?

Conclusive of what is written

Tongues have been bitten

Ears have bled from what was said

Blistered wounds raised

Eyes amazed

Though cannot praise

The phase of negative craze

That are present

These days

****

EMOTIONS

Whatever state of being you are in now is directly linked to what you are thinking, feeling, and imagining. So why not think, feel, and imagine freely flowing cells — free from harmful substances (bacteria, viruses, heavy metals, sensitivities), negative thoughts, feelings, and actions? It may take effort to push through, but positive habits can eventually take over and start working with you in your healing journey.

Prayers and affirmations are amazingly effective. You can use something you already know or have read somewhere that really resonates with you, or you can create your own. Creating your own prayer or affirmation will give it a personal touch by using words that have a greater potential to connect with your inner self.

Choose or create one statement, one sentence. There may be a lot you want to change, but keeping it short and sweet makes it easier to remember and repeat multiple times throughout the day. That's doable, right? So, what is your statement? What is your sentence? What is your affirmation? You can create as many as you want, but pick no more than three to start with – you can say one when you wake up, one at midday, and one before going to bed. You can also repeat them throughout the day.

One of my statements is: *"My red blood cells are whole, healthy, and happy."* As I say this, I automatically visualize red blood cells in their non-sickled form, traveling through my veins with ease. Injecting affirmations into your subconscious mind will help you develop resistance to feeling miserable. Research has found a high prevalence of depression in people with sickle cell disease, which ultimately decreases quality of life. Interestingly enough, depressed patients also report more frequent episodes.

The way you feel directly affects the way your cells vibrate and act. Poor emotional health can weaken the immune system (which we absolutely cannot afford), decrease the function of our organs and systems, and increase our susceptibility to infection. Whenever an uneasy emotion arises, identify why you may be feeling that way and adjust your mental attitude and focus accordingly.

Redirecting negative energy into a positive thought can improve how oxygen circulates through your body (relieving tension) for the effective functioning of your red blood cells, enabling them to last as long as possible without dying off even more prematurely than they already do. When adjusting our emotional frequency, we must be willing and able. The very fact that you are reading this book proves that you are willing and able.

MEDITATION

"You have power over your mind, not outside events. Realize this, and you will find strength."

– Marcus Aurelius

Meditation is not just a tool for relaxation; it's a pathway to deeper healing of both body and mind. When we bring our attention to the breath, a word, or a simple image, we begin to melt the layers of stress, fear, and discomfort that usually fuel both physical pain and emotional unrest. Research published in the *Journal of Neuroscience* by Fadel Zeidan[1] shows that meditation can reduce the perception of pain by

---

[1] https://pubmed.ncbi.nlm.nih.gov/21471390/

up to 40% and decrease activity in the brain's pain centers by nearly 60%.

Furthermore, a systematic review[2] in 2024 also found that:

- Mindfulness-Based Stress Reduction (MBSR) enhances brain regions related to emotional processing and sensory perception.

- It improves psychological outcomes like anxiety and depression.

- It exhibits unique mechanisms of pain reduction compared to a placebo.

When faced with the initial stages of a sickle cell episode, more often than not, our emotions descend into negativity. Our thoughts scan the endless possibilities of how the upcoming days will look if things don't improve soon. These uneasy feelings are natural, but the vibrations we experience can signal internal distress. This may then ultimately increase our pain perception, leading to a potential extreme crisis. I'm not saying that engaging in mindfulness or meditation will prevent you from having an extreme episode, but it can drastically ease the whole experience if you do. Instead of focusing on unfavorable outcomes and physical discomfort, be mindful and accepting of the unpredictability of your condition. Take hold of the situation. Take hold of

---

[2] https://pubmed.ncbi.nlm.nih.gov/39595177/

the perspective of moving through another victory with serenity, rather than only preparing for the worst with hostility. As Bruce Lipton stated,

"Beliefs and thoughts alter cells in your body. Each of our cells is a living entity, and the main thing that influences them is our blood. If I open my eyes in the morning and someone I deeply care about is in front of me, my perception causes a release of oxytocin, dopamine, and growth hormones – all of which encourage the growth and health of my cells. But if I see a saber-tooth tiger, I'm going to release stress hormones, which change the cells to a protection mode. People need to realize that their thoughts are more primary than their genes, because the environment, which is influenced by our thoughts, controls the genes."

– Bruce Lipton

Meditation does not ask us to empty the mind, but to become more intimate with it. Whatever we give our focused attention to—whether a healing thought, a word, or a peaceful image—grows stronger within us. If you feel unsure where to start, simply return to a phrase or theme from the earlier chapters that deeply resonated with you. You might also hold a single word in your mind, such as *joy, strength,* or *courage.* This repetitive focus, known as *mantra meditation,* can be practiced throughout the day—while walking, resting, or especially before sleep, when the subconscious is more receptive to healing impressions.

Playing music or sounds (such as soothing instrumentals, binaural beats, or solfeggio frequencies) while meditating helps me enter a deeper, more comfortable space within and enhances the experience. Select a specific sound (various frequencies have different meanings) and enter a comfortable space. Turn off all other electronics, and focus your mind by taking slow, deep breaths.

You can use the exercise in Chapter 4. Once you reach your maximum number of deep breaths (up to 10, for instance), return to your regular breathing pattern. Focus your mind on one of the personal affirmations you've developed and continue to repeat it rhythmically. Visualize your veins as robust and healthy, providing oxygen and nourishment to all of your organs and systems. Visualize the cells flowing through your veins without blockages, without struggle, reaching where they need to be. Your bone marrow is keeping up the pace by producing more red blood cells. Your oxygen levels are increasing. Your body is healing. *So shall it be.*

This simple meditation can be personalized to suit your current condition, although the steps remain the same. Setting time for meditation is not about *finding* the time but *making* the time. You can meditate at any time, day or night. Start with at least four times per week, eventually making it a daily habit. There's time for everything; we just need to prioritize and clarify what we truly need. Meditation benefits not only your body but also your mind. Falling asleep and/or waking up to something positive, like this, can impress both your subconscious and conscious minds, manifesting a change in frequency within your body — one that can dramatically affect your health.

At times, messages (insightful impressions on the mind) can surface during meditation. They may come from a vision, a thought, a dream, or just a personal longing. Record these messages. They've come to you for a reason. Gain a deeper understanding and act on these messages to achieve greater health and longevity.

MINDFULNESS

Mindfulness is one of those quiet things that can profoundly change how we navigate life. It's about being fully present and not weighed down by old memories, future worries, beliefs, or judgments. Just here. Just now. Can you sit in this moment without needing to change it, without rushing to label it? Try it out, even if it's just for a few deep breaths.

Mindfulness isn't about sitting still or clearing your mind. It's about paying attention to your thoughts, your body, and the world around you, and choosing to be fully present within your own life.

It's a lot like breathwork. Normally, we breathe without thinking. But when we slow down and consciously guide each inhale and exhale, everything shifts. The same goes for mindfulness. Instead of running on autopilot, going through routines without even noticing, we actually *live* our lives. Even simple things like folding laundry, cooking a meal, or walking outside feel different when you're really *there* for them.

Shown to literally change the structure of the brain, mindfulness strengthens parts that support memory, learning, and emotional balance, while calming down areas that react to stress and fear.[3] Over time, mindfulness stops feeling like just another practice. It becomes a way of living—clearer, more real.

On the emotional side, mindfulness builds resilience. Living with sickle cell often comes with feelings of anxiety, sadness, or frustration. Mindfulness doesn't erase these feelings, but it helps you hold them with more consideration and less overwhelm. When you're mindful, you're no longer just reacting to every spike of pain or fatigue; you're tuning into your body's needs with more compassion and insight. You start to notice earlier when your body asks for rest, hydration, movement, or emotional support, which can help prevent crises or lessen their severity. It won't make the pain disappear, but it can certainly shift your relationship with it, allowing you to live with more presence, more strength, and more peace, even on the toughest days.

---

[3] https://www.nature.com/articles/nrn3916

Mindfulness is a powerful tool for living with sickle cell anemia, both physically and emotionally. We often experience unpredictable pain episodes, fatigue, and emotional ups and downs. Mindfulness helps by teaching the body and mind how to respond rather than react to these challenges. Instead of the body being stuck in a cycle of tension, fear, and pain, mindfulness creates space. Space to breathe through pain, to soften into the present moment, even when it's hard.

Meditation can also have surprising benefits and the power to engulf you in the process of moving your body towards greater awareness. Whether you've tried meditation in the past or are new to the concept of tapping into your subconscious, it is a phenomenal therapeutic practice that calms the mind and simultaneously taps into the healing capabilities of your own body.

MINDFULNESS MOMENT:

Wherever you are, pause for just 60 seconds.

Take a slow, deep breath in... and let it go gently.

Now, notice:

- What sounds do you hear around you?

- What sensations can you feel in your body—tightness, warmth, tension, ease?

- What emotion is lightly sitting with you right now, without needing to fix it or change it?

Stay curious.

You don't have to do anything special. Just notice.

This is mindfulness.

REDUCED ENVIRONMENTAL STIMULATION THERAPY

Another beautiful way to reconnect with ourselves, nurture cellular healing, soothe pain, and relax deeply into the body is through flotation, also known as *reduced environmental stimulation therapy*, *float tank*, or *sensory deprivation chamber*. These tanks are filled with tepid water saturated with over 1,000 pounds of Epsom salts. Known for reducing inflammation and pain, the salts allow the body to become effortlessly buoyant, weightless, and still. Additionally, freed from the pull of gravity and external stimulation, the nervous system is given a rare chance to rest at an optimal level.

Research has shown that floating can reduce cortisol levels, ease chronic pain, and enhance mental clarity by shifting the brain into a deeply restorative theta wave state, similar to that of deep meditation and early sleep.[4] During this stillness, the mind has the opportunity to release old

---

[4] https://pmc.ncbi.nlm.nih.gov/articles/PMC5796691/

tension patterns, allowing both emotional and physical healing to take place naturally.

A one-hour float session has been proven to have the same benefits as an 8-hour restful sleep, calming the nervous system and enhancing your body's natural ability to heal. If you ever try this out for yourself, remember to ask for a tank that has the warmest temperature. Even though they are usually all at room temperature, I've always asked if there is one slightly warmer than the rest, so I don't eventually get too cold in there. After all, it lasts about an hour. Since this is water, not nitrogen gas like in cryotherapy sessions, be mindful of not getting to the point of shivering or feeling cold once you're in there. When you get out, the evaporation of water can make the body cooler, which can lead to disaster and counteract the healing you were trying to achieve in the first place. A nice, warm shower right after you're out of the chamber is helpful for removing salt and dead skin. Then, a more comfortable, steamy one at home does the trick.

If you have access to a float center, consider treating yourself to a full sensory float experience. If not, you can recreate a smaller version at home by filling your bathtub with approximately 2 cups of Epsom salts for every gallon (about 4 liters) of water. Adding essential oils like frankincense, rosemary, lavender, or camphor can enhance the therapeutic benefits. Even a simple soak can be a doorway back to yourself—into that sacred space where healing begins, not by force, but by surrender.

SLEEP

To enhance your willingness and ability to function optimally, allow yourself to take the rest you need. This is vital. Have you ever noticed that whenever you are sleep-deprived, you feel, think, or act differently? Well, of course! How can you truly be yourself if you're deprived of the natural healing process your body requires to survive? Sleep helps you heal. Not only sleep, but rest as much as you can.

I know many of you warriors out there may want to do things on your own and push through in order to sustain your life's routines. That's perfectly understandable. Just remember that sometimes pushing too far can backfire. Sleep is a way to significantly enhance your mental well-being with sufficient rest and relaxation. Don't neglect one of the easiest forms of healing available to you.

It's okay to delegate household chores to other family members or to those who are willing to help. You don't need to carry everything on your shoulders. You have lovely people around you who would be more than happy to help. And if you're on your own, you're the only one you need to look after, so embrace that.

When you get the necessary rest and your mental state is rejuvenated, you will feel clearer about the daily decisions you make, especially those related to your health.

Take my client, Shauna, for example. She was so frustrated with all the responsibilities of her daily routine.

Feeling stressed only aggravated how she felt. Every day was a repeat of this same frustration and stress. When she realized that her cyclical thought patterns were draining her energy, she decided to make a change.

Once she had her priorities straight, she altered some things. She started only cooking three or four days per week, allowing her to put aside food for the days she didn't cook. She also delegated household responsibilities to her daughters. All of this allowed her to increase her sleep from approximately five hours per night to seven hours most nights.

This made a huge change in the way she felt about herself. Her moods were better, which was reflected in her higher energy levels and overall sense of well-being. She noticed fewer mild episodes than she used to, which was great for her and her family.

As the Dalai Lama said, *"Sleep is the best meditation."*

It may feel selfish to take a nap, or you may worry that you'll seem lazy. However, taking the time to rest can create a positive environment for your blood cells to flow calmly, rather than being agitated by your thoughts and emotions. You, and only you, can ensure that you are getting the proper amount of sleep you need.

RELEASING NEGATIVITY

What are some ways you've released stress in the past? Did you rest or sleep? Did you exercise? Take a walk? Talk to someone? Write? Any of these can guide you toward a better state of mind. Personally, I like to write. Writing poetry about various issues has gotten me through some rough times. It is a way for me to express my experiences, which allows me to gain strength to move forward and face the next challenge.

Repeating and visualizing empowering words and truly believing that you are blessed in every way can move you towards better outcomes. Although at times, the mental stress and pain of sickle cell disease can be unbearable, you can work towards refocusing your mind on what you really want for yourself.

You don't always have to accept what is being fed to you by the medical profession alone. Know you are worth more than submitting to that. You possess a powerful mental ability to direct your body towards massive healing through what you know to be true for you. Face it, we know our own bodies best since we've been living in them since birth.

Yes, health care professionals can offer research-based recommendations based on your symptoms and past health experiences, but you are the one making the ultimate decision. Make the proper choice for yourself based not only

on what's in the books, but also on what you can manifest
through your own desire for health.

****

<u>POWER WITHIN</u>

Insanity to let you get the best of me

And brainwash this mind

To a minute piece of grain

Either you have a corrupt plan

Or I'm just walking in the wrong lane

Must be

The bane of your presence to lead others astray

That causes detrimental repercussions

To your spirit

By far thou dost revere it

The fact that I am a strong blessed woman

On a mission

A mission that excludes people like you

Who like to go deep

Surely, not mentally deep,

But deep within your spiritual realm

Of non-existence

Compared to my co-existence

With this universe of life

Assume no dominance in my space

For my space must replace

Pride with grace

Disloyalty with devotion

Egoism to freedom

Greed with abundance and wealth

Want with purpose

Segregation with unity

And disease with purity

This is me

My soul who speaks

Let the body retreat

While the soul confronts to teach

Teach those who are willing to learn

Are on the verge of destruction

And those who are already there

Why care?

This is the place in which we reside

Can't hide and see

Wherever you run to, there you will be.

I play no devil's advocate to be happy in living a lie

For the vibrations of these communications

Releases my frustrations within this empty nation

Empty like the fall branches of a maple tree

Naked with no substance

Bare and tainted

Like the minds of those who waste it

Covered with the darkness of inner lack

Train to stay on track and fight back

To face the facts

Get off the high that makes you just get by and

Use that energy to control

How your spirit controls you

Now from out of one vessel

Can flow the necessities of all mankind

Eradicate the social conspiracies

That verbalize that now is not the time

For time is but a breath of air

That fuels our self with life

Yet I live among the dead

Among the really breathing, but not breathing real.

As you come to the place of over-standing,

Realize that the truth has been told

A spark you must behold

And wisdom is only for the selected

A shame to see it rejected

And placed below the rank of being elected

My soul aches

Though it cannot break the intensity

The authority of this deep inner strength

One that binds the accumulation of the weak

Endures the everlasting blows of the inevitable

Ever-changing yet always the same

Strive for private principle-centered victories

At the mercy of

The power within

The power within cannot be fed from the material

Confusing the illusion of what is really seen

It hungers for the ethereal

For what cannot be seen

So disperse, you fiend

And for those who may not comprehend, may ask,

"Well, Essense, what do you mean?"

Then my response is…

Seek and you shall find,

For these words are not only for the mind

I'm brought up and livin' in sin,

There's toxic residues

Thickening underneath my skin

To look through these worldly visions

Where and how shall we begin?

By the mighty, authentic, spiritual gift of…

The power within

Chapter 9
Handling Crises Like a Pro: Before, During, and After an Episode

So here it is. You're in pain. You're home alone, with no one available to help. If you experience a crisis at home, you may have a greater chance of healing more rapidly without the additional stress of hospitalization. So, what do you do?

If possible, gather as many supplies as you can to keep by your side, such as medications, water, a heating pad, and a phone. Do what you know works for you, take your meds, settle in, and hope for the best.

One of the most frustrating things we face is that so few people will ever understand the extent of energy needed to bear the pain of an intense sickle cell episode. Once in a while, you may want to push through and continue with your daily routine. You know your body best.

As you continue to progress through the episode, you'll know what you need to do. Depending on the severity, it can disrupt the very essence of who you are. Remember, you are so strong. Think about your intentions in life. Yes, your intentions. If you're focused on how much the pain is affecting you at this point, you're fueling the fire. As difficult as it may be, concentrating on your intentions, passions, purpose, and the lessons you've learned over the years will redirect your energy from the excruciating pain.

It's so easy to become overwhelmingly bitter and frustrated, but instead, use this episode as an opportunity to become stronger and more positive, to shift the frequencies of your internal vibrations. In turn, this will keep you more centered amidst the massive disruption and turmoil going on within your veins. This is your mental power at work. Your body may have already called the shots, but you can still protect yourself against further damage by calling in the army of your mind.

As you already know, this too shall pass. Keep your mind on your work, your family, and your responsibilities. Seek to maintain calmness through the unbearable torture. Yes, there may be painful twitches, squirms, screams, and painful rants. I truly understand. But just as swimming against the current exhausts the body while floating allows it to move with ease, it's going to take more energy to try and fight the pain and discomfort rather than to surrender to your positive mind.

Turning your attention to your breath may help you to take slower, deeper inhalations and exhalations from the diaphragm, rather than shallow breathing from the chest. Oxygen is vital here.

Most of us only surrender to the hospital as a "last resort." This is a totally valid choice if there are no other significant issues you may be experiencing, for example, regular transfusions, dialysis, chronic symptoms, or additional medical conditions. These have the potential to increase your body's sensitivity, and in many cases, medical assistance would be the only way to rapidly restore homeostasis within your cells, veins, organs, and systems.

DURING AN EPISODE

If you don't have one already, create a plan of action for when a severe crisis arises – those crippling events that leave you quite helpless and dependent on others. Think ahead to what your children and other loved ones may experience during these times. We should have these discussions beforehand so that all parties involved can be prepared at any time.

Who will take you to the hospital if necessary? Who will take care of your children and other personal responsibilities when you're not home? Once all this has been established, your mind should be clear enough to move forward with getting well. You matter most. It's important not to rush through the pain. It's great to have the mentality that you must come first. Getting well to the best of your ability is the main focus here, not all the other responsibilities and obligations that are waiting for you.

The less energy you need to exert during your crisis, the more energy you will have available when you emerge from it. There have been instances where I would push through the pain because my "mommy mentality" told me I had to go to work to take care of my son. He has helped me develop one of the most critical aspects of living with sickle cell – the drive to continue. He has kept my spirits higher than anyone else. I really don't know where I would be today without the joy he brings. I am blessed by his natural efforts to help get me well on those fateful days when I feel like I have no hope.

Who does this for you? Being surrounded by the right person or group of people can engulf you with positive energy, much like laughter does. Do yourself a favor and smile. Laugh. A genuine one that creases the corners of your eyes. Yes, that kind of laugh and smile. Fill those cells of yours with the joy they need to be healthy and survive. Fill yourself with the happiness you are meant to have, live, and enjoy.

YOUR JOY

Do what you love. Go to a place where you can feel overwhelmingly content. And if that's not possible because of physical constraints, remember that you are already there. You're already in that place of bliss and solitude; it's only your body blocking you from feeling that way. What makes it easier is envisioning your bliss. Envision your purpose. Just as it is with our traumas, you were meant to learn from, live through, and break through the genetic barriers you were born with.

Unlike a vast percentage of the population, we must learn our way not only through life itself, but also through the condition we were given. Finding our true joy can switch those cellular electromagnetic frequencies. It may come from spending time with a family member, friend, colleague, or someone else, or from doing something that brings a genuine, true element of joy.

When you're going through a crisis, you can recover more quickly by finding peace, joy, happiness, exuberance, passion, strength, enlightenment, and greatness, rather than being angry, frustrated, hopeless, saddened, or even depressed (which is easy to feel but obviously negative). It takes effort to redirect our thought processes in such situations, but you do have the time. Rest. Hydrate. Breathe. Focus your thoughts. It is only in your best interest to help your body recuperate as soon as possible.

Take this opportunity to refocus and regroup. You do not need to treat your episode as "just another one that inevitably had to happen." Ask yourself: What led to it? Were you involved in a situation that swayed you from your genuine life path? Did you eat or drink something that aggravated you at the cellular level? What did you do or think? What is this really about?

It's not always just another crisis. Could this be a way for your body to tell you that something needs to change, just like if you had an allergy? Since this is the DNA we were given, our environment constantly alters our natural internal mechanisms to adapt. Sickle cell may have developed as an adaptation response connected to malaria. Our new adaptation response is influenced by many external factors, which have led us to look more within. Are you still with me here? This adaptation response is adversely affected by the numerous external factors that impact the mechanism within. Sickle cell may affect one person much differently than someone else diagnosed with the same condition. Since this is the case, recognizing and recording patterns is essential. We'll explore this more in Chapter 10.

THE AFTERMATH

What we face here is almost like a battle within our own bodies, and we have the potential to win this battle one step at a time. Embracing joy in the midst of turmoil and excruciating pain may just be the armor you need. As you begin to feel well enough to integrate more and more principles from this book into your daily routine, don't forget about what you just went through during this crisis. What did you learn in that state? We can always gain insight from our internal cellular insufficiency.

If you were able to get through the pain yet again, let it not be in vain. Embrace and accept what your body is trying to tell you, because everything we endure in this life has a purpose. It just *is*. The purpose of a sneeze is to quickly clear the nose and throat of an irritant that has had a chance to enter our passageways. Sickle cell is undoubtedly more complicated, of course, but we must still embrace the same natural law of cause and effect: *for every action, there is a reaction.*

In our case, eliminating the irritant means flushing out the veins by increasing oxygen and circulation for our red blood cells. The body is constantly swaying towards and away from balance, trying – even without our conscious effort – to maintain balance in order to function optimally. If our bodies do this without our conscious effort, what if we were to make a conscious effort? What greater effect could this cause?

FROM TORTURE TO NURTURE

Nurture yourself. Assist the temple you were given with the necessary attention it deserves. After an episode, and even during, or ideally as much as possible, including when you're feeling your best, fuel yourself with foods, liquids, people, thoughts, and environments that will nurture a body recovering from illness. Don't like the taste of certain natural foods or fresh juices? Experiment with different combinations and let your taste buds guide you! This is about wanting the best for yourself so you can be more present for your family, your work, and, most importantly, for yourself.

This is not a joke. If you were faced with a major challenge in your life (as if sickle cell itself isn't one), you would definitely do whatever it took to get through that. Sickle cell *is* a major challenge. It's not something that just happens along our life journey. It's something that was passed on to us, and we must now overcome it. Do not pass this on to the next generation without awareness. Educate your children and potential partners about your status. Take this as seriously as any other life-defining situation or lesson.

Fuel your body. Take care of it. It's taking care of you every single day. Since our subconscious teaches our conscious minds, it is important to feed our subconscious with the positive healing power it was meant to have. This reciprocates. The law of attraction and vibration states that like attracts like, and people receive the energy they project.

****

<u>I SHALL RISE</u>

Make way today 'cause my vivid dreams will rise above

There are

Clear explanations with destinations

Reaching the level of expectation

For my divine manifestation

That of peace, light, honor, and glory

An immaculate piece of this life

Making the future, present, and history

Shedding the old to unfold my new testimony

Embarking on a lasting impression

Like Nubian ancestry

A mastery

In the science of esoteric living

Giving

Way for my new beginning

Sinning

Not at the soul spiritual level of conscience, but

Aren't I a tad glad that I am human?

Assuming but not abusing, losing sight

Of why I am here

My eyes continue to clear

And I increasingly fear the

Sensei of my home

You may call it Earth

But I, the entire Universe

As limitless as the skies

From my eyes

The emancipation loosens the cry

Try

Not to overlook the concept of growth

'Cause ultimately there is no measure in size

The lessons of the wise

Which is why

I shall rise

There has been

A picture painted legacy of me

A masterpiece of a divine design

As unique and different each cell of the way

Needless to say

Upon concentration...

Money, luck, protection, courage, energy, divination

Is what my goal is

A tiger's eye

Holding the crystal close

I propose to my soul and

The celestial gods and goddesses

Who have pulled me through

There ain't nothin' I can do

Than to let it take over and allow me to rise

I'm so determined, I'm focusized

Breaking through the barriers

Like a Leo in the first house

As quiet as a mouse

And vibrant like Venus in heat

Allow me to take the seat

Crowned as Essense

The founder of a new era complete and concrete

So glad you and I can meet and greet

The intersection upon my feet

In the attempt of deciding on which way to go

I continue to flow to

Let you know

Where I have gained or lost sight

Within each word that I unite

Feeling the electrical currents through my dendrites

There is nothing orally right that I refuse to invite

It's in my nature to internalize

To devise at my surprise

My prophetic

Poetic

Karmic

Classic ability

To rise

Chapter 10
Embrace the Process: Track Your Wellness Milestones

Tracking your progress will help you pinpoint triggers you may not have correlated with pain before. For instance, maybe you and your family have been eating the same meals together for years. But what if one of those regular meals has been aggravating your symptoms and condition without you realizing it? Once certain symptoms such as irritability or fatigue become part of our daily routine, we may say things like, *"Oh, I always feel like that,"* or *"That's normal for me."* Yes, I understand sickle cell is often associated with certain symptoms, but some of these symptoms can be drastically reduced, or even avoided, if we are mindful enough.

This book can offer you a great deal of helpful recommendations, but if you're just doing what you think is right for you without a way to measure your progress, how will you know if what you're doing is working? There will be both subtle and more noticeable changes when you are working towards optimal health. Ask yourself: What changes do I feel in my emotions? Has the duration or intensity of my pain episodes changed? What was I doing when my crisis started?

You'll also want to jot down things like what foods you had eaten and how much water you were drinking, along with any stressors and responses (physical, emotional, mental) to those stressors. When information is recorded correctly, you can always look back and discover advantageous patterns, or those that you should do away with because they don't serve you. Tracking these alterations lets you create the most result-driven expectations you desire out of this illness.

Don't make it hard to do what is easy (even though it may seem tedious at first). To truly achieve your desired health outcomes, you must be willing to approach things differently and move closer to the results you desire. Recording health notes in my calendar or journal allows me to go back and see what may have accelerated an imbalance internally, aggravating my symptoms. This strategy has been very beneficial not only for me, but also for my clients.

Your mission? Start with these headings, and then create your own personalized tracking chart by adding any other information that is specific to you:

- Date

- Food Journal (portion sizes of food items and non-food items)

- Supplements

- Cravings (specific food item, or by taste–sweet, salty, sour, etc.)

- Total Water Intake

- Bowel Movements (number of times per day, color, size, and consistency–e.g., 2, light brown, long, firm)

- Pain Intensity (scale from 1-10)

- Time of Pain Onset

- Location & Level of Pain

- Medication Taken (prescription and over-the-counter)

- Energy Level (scale from 1-10)

- Exercise (type, duration)

- Stress Level (1-10)

- Mood/Emotion

- Productivity (ability to perform work-related and non-work-related activities)

THREE-DAY EXAMPLE:

	Day 1	Day 2	Day 3
Date			
Food Journal	Breakfast: Cornmeal and oats porridge	Breakfast: Toast with hummus, one apple	Breakfast: Smoothie, toast with hummus
	Lunch: Mixed bean salad, hummus, and rice cakes (2) fermented protein smoothie	Lunch: Sandwich, chips, soda	Lunch: Vegetable soup, tuna sandwich, water
	Dinner: Mixed vegetables (stir-fried), baked salmon	Dinner: Baked sweet potato, bean salad	Dinner: Stir-fry shrimp and rice, vegetables
Supplements	Vitamin C 1,500, B complex 100mg, Vitamin D 3,000,	Probiotic, B complex 100mg, vitamin D 3,000, vitamin C	Probiotic, B complex 100mg, vitamin D 3,000, vitamin C

	Super Enzymes w/meals Fermented protein smoothie: hemp, rice, pea protein, fermented l-glutamine, sea vegetables mix (spirulina, Irish moss, chlorella, dulse, etc.), sunflower seed butter, banana, mixed berries	1,500 Fermented protein smoothie: hemp, rice, pea protein, fermented l-glutamine, sea vegetables mix (spirulina, Irish moss, chlorella, dulse, etc.), sunflower seed butter, banana, mixed berries	1,500 Fermented protein smoothie: hemp, rice, pea protein, fermented l-glutamine, sea vegetables mix (spirulina, Irish moss, chlorella, dulse, etc.), sunflower seed butter, banana, mixed berries
Cravings	None	Sweet	None
Total Water Intake	2L, with chlorophyll	2.5L, with chlorophyll	2L, with chlorophyll
Bowel Movements	2	2	3
Pain intensity (1-10)	5	6	7

Time of pain onset	2 pm	All day	All day
Location of pain	Right wrist	Right wrist and arm	Right wrist and arm
Medication Taken	None	Advil Extra Strength, two capsules (2x)	Advil Extra Strength, two capsules (2x)
Energy Level (1-10)	7	6	4
Exercise	None	None	None
Stress Level (1-10)	5	5	8
Mood/Emotion	Happy	Content	Sad
Female Cycle	Day 3 of Menses	Day 4 of Menses	Day 5 of Menses
Productivity	8	6	4

PRACTICE MAKES PROGRESS

No one is perfect by any means, though we are all perfect in our own unique way. Understanding your triggers is very helpful in this process. Some triggers may not be obvious, which is why charting can prove to be highly beneficial if you stick with it. Missing a day or two of charting may not seem like a significant issue, but remember that everything we do physically, emotionally, mentally, and spiritually has consequences, whether beneficial or not. When you eat or drink something out of the ordinary, or respond with an emotion to a particular experience, it can significantly impact the type of day you have, which can ultimately boost or drain your energy. Seeking patterns in these areas can help you understand how your body responds to specific situations.

Reflection is the mother of wisdom. Reflect on your completed chart entries from time to time, perhaps at the end of each week and month. This will make it easier to identify areas where you may not have performed well, notice any habits, and make any necessary adjustments. You may be surprised at what you find!

Mastering yourself is true power. Your body communicates with you every day, at every moment. Are you listening? Are you paying attention to those cues? Or are you too caught up in everyday life? Your body will thank you once you begin to listen to it and make the changes required for a healthier well-being.

The connection between your needs and wants plays a significant role here. When you are focused on what you *want*, you push yourself further away from what you really *need*. You want to get well, you want to be pain-free, you *want*, you *want*, you *want*. But what are you willing to *do*? Shift that language: *I will track my progress to get well. I will take the necessary steps to enhance my health and have the energy to take care of myself and my family.*

When you put it in this perspective, then your needs become much more realistic because the *"why"* is there. Wanting is dreaming. Needing means focusing your mind on what will truly meet those needs, and then finding a way to do so. Your goal is to prevent future episodes or lessen their duration and intensity by realizing what you can do differently.

Tracking should not feel like a chore. It should become part of your everyday routine, just like brushing your teeth. Make it a natural part of your routine to take care of yourself. Acknowledge the wisdom and power within. Do not leave your well-being *solely* in the hands of health care providers who are trained with protocols that may or may not be in the best interest of your true health. Listening to and understanding your unique body is not something that a physician will be able to do for you. Focus on taking care of yourself to make informed choices for the most favorable outcomes.

On a scale from 1-10, how committed are you to taking the steps to gain and improve the vitality you were meant to have? This will not work if you don't do the work. So what is your number? Committing to this doesn't mean reading these words; it means putting them into practice. One step at a time. That's all it takes. Along with your symptoms, record your foods and other activities, as well as your expectations, in your charting process. You're not only tracking; you are also manifesting.

Once you're in the habit of tracking your progress, whether once a day or multiple times throughout the day, it will provide both you and your healthcare provider with the information needed to adjust your treatment protocol if necessary. It allows you to deepen your connection to what you truly need. As committed as physicians, nurses, and researchers are to furthering and applying their knowledge to help us, we must be even more committed to our own recovery, healing, and wellness.

AWAY FROM THE CONVENTIONAL

On a percentage scale from 0-100%, where would you rate yourself in terms of your medical involvement? As vital as treatment can be for many, it often presents serious implications. Again, you know your body best. By no means am I suggesting you stop any treatment you are currently under. You know what is best for you. What I am saying is that the body and cells can only recover under the most favorable circumstances. Once this homeostasis is disrupted, it takes significantly more energy for the body to adjust and adapt to the substances intended to treat it.

Recognizing patterns on your own gives you the insight to make beneficial decisions for your healthcare and integrate these practices into your current standard of care. As you apply the strategies in this book and track your progress over time, you should begin to notice improvement in your symptoms. The goal here is to decrease the percentage of medical care necessary to control your condition.

It's one thing to simply take the necessary steps to strengthen your system and provide your cells with the best possible environment to function. But knowing the reasons behind your symptoms, behind those dreadful attacks, and having an overview recorded on paper gives you a clear guide of what needs to be adjusted. Nutrition is not the only factor. It could be anything in your daily routine, such as your emotions, your relationships, your thinking patterns, your attitude towards change, your desire to get the most out of life, etc. Only *you* can control these things.

We are constantly receiving clues from our bodies, but we often get so distracted by other issues that we miss them. Without the proof of your tracking record, you have no way of knowing what may truly be happening or how to make adjustments and progress. You may have adapted to a state you call "normal," but you do not have to surrender to it. Commit yourself to knowing what you really need in all aspects of your life, because everything that happens outside of you affects the inside of you, and vice versa. Anything that happens externally sends signals at the cellular level, which affects the red blood cells and, subsequently, the oxygen supply. Healing starts within, so that it can manifest outwards.

Chapter 11
Keep Moving Forward: Thriving Beyond Sickle Cell

I'm sure there have been instances in your life where you needed to adapt. If you have to take sick time off work, for example, it affects your finances, your personal duties, and family responsibilities because your ability to attend to these things may be limited. The inevitable happens. We have no choice but to adjust and adapt when needed. Of course, situations may arise that are beyond our control, but there are things we can certainly change, and you have the power to do so. You have the power to say, "Enough is enough," and nurture yourself so that not everything is just left up to chance.

Have you ever been so excited to do something and then, after a few days, weeks, or months, you fall off? Take exercise, for instance. I love the feeling I get after a good workout. I tend to have spurts of getting a good schedule going, then life happens. Either I get caught up with responsibilities, or I stop because I feel something coming on and want to avoid aggravating what could lead to an intense episode.

But when I stop exercising, I just end up feeling drained and more susceptible to illness. It's important that I start again to get the most out of my health. When you're in a state of less pain, you have no excuse not to do the best you can to get the most out of your body. Our muscles weaken if they are not used regularly. Just as a plant withers without being nurtured, your body will wither as well and will take much longer to reverse the symptoms you experience. Similarly, if we don't focus on our goals, we lose our will to manifest them as a reality.

This has a particular importance for sickle cell patients because every time we experience an episode, damage is done to our muscles, bones, and organs. It affects our entire being. Myonecrosis is already a complication, so why not take a proactive approach to help lessen its negative effects? We must accept that complications may happen, and still work to reduce their chances. Prevention is better than cure.

It does take effort. Are you willing to do what it takes? Are you willing to sacrifice the routine you've been used to all these years? Are you willing to get out of your comfort zone? Are you ready to make your health a priority, not only for yourself, but also for those who depend on you? For your own sanity? For your future?

It's easy to get discouraged, especially when dealing with such a crippling condition. I totally acknowledge this. It may be helpful to start today by becoming clear on how you see yourself in 1, 5, 10, or 20 years in terms of your health. How will you make yourself better today? What will you do differently? What will be your new habits? You have the tools. Take the necessary steps along the way with no guilt or judgment. You only fail if you don't start at all.

Look at the number of obstacles you've had to pave through to get to where you are now. You are a warrior! Use that spirit to further your health. There will always be obstacles. It's about getting over them with as minimal effort as possible. This requires that soldier spirit you already have. It's a shame that sickle cell warriors aren't recognized enough for their strength and resilience. Having an amazing support system provides the fuel for us to move further along our journey, but it's ultimately up to us to take the steps toward greater health and wellness. Own it. You deserve it.

When you notice that you're not doing your tracking, or taking in enough fluids, or feeling too fatigued to initiate anything, harness that state of being and listen. Your body is trying to tell you something. This is not how you're supposed to feel. Just because you've been diagnosed with sickle cell doesn't mean all symptoms are an excuse not to act. There's something that needs to change and be adjusted. You know what you're doing and not doing. Therefore, make the necessary changes.

Again, why make it hard to do what is easy? For the most part, it's just deciding to make yourself a priority and reap the benefits of better health and less pain. When things get worse, there's a reason. When turmoil arises within your cells, there's a reason. Discovering that reason can lead you to a much more productive and joyous life, enabling you to do the little things we all take for granted.

Being happy is a choice, yes. But being grateful to be alive should be a fact. Use this fact to propel yourself into a state of unshakeable dedication to your health and wellbeing. Work with your health care provider to understand how your unique body functions, guiding you to a deeper understanding of yourself and how your body reacts to inner and outer influences. Finding the best remedy to take isn't always the answer. It is a whole lifestyle. You can do this. Your loved ones are counting on you. So am I.

ONE STEP AT A TIME

Since sickle cell is a condition that you don't just develop, it's not like taking a pill will make it feel better. Hydroxyurea may be an option, along with others currently in trial, but sickle cell disease doesn't go away unless you've undergone an invasive procedure, such as a bone marrow transplant, stem cell transplant, or Exa-Cel (CRISPR gene editing treatment). It is up to us to overcome our obstacles even more than we have been doing on a day-to-day basis. Accelerate this by recognizing your worth and purpose. How do you see yourself when you finally have optimal energy levels and fewer attacks? Visualize yourself in this state.

If you really don't think this could be a reality, then stop reading. If you don't believe in your potential, you will not succeed. You won't make the effort necessary to make progress. You will only know if you do the work and remain consistent. Decide to habitually adapt one thing at a time until it becomes second nature, such as always having water with you, proper supplementation, eating right (at least 80% of the time), practicing deep breathing, engaging in effective exercise, etc. These habits will lead you toward a healthier body, mind, and spirit – a healthier you.

So, what one step will you take today to further your health goals? Rushing to try and incorporate everything too soon will only lead to disappointment. You will only take the necessary steps when you have the motivation. It's like telling a child "no." Children need a reason not to do something, or they'll just want to do the opposite of what you tell them. If you've read this far, you know why I'm asking you to do these things. You have the reason. You have the courage. Take action. Become who you were undoubtedly meant to be, despite your challenges, despite the unpredictability.

This healing process requires your focus and attention. Whenever you start something new, there's always going to be some sort of resistance and new symptoms that may arise. Whether physical, emotional, or mental, something will change. This is expected. Take these adjustments seriously and record them on your tracking sheet. Take a proactive approach to your health. Use the results of your medical exams and sensitivity tests to adjust your routine and methods as needed, in consultation with your healthcare provider or nutritionist.

Tracking your progress and getting more in tune with your body – to its strengths and weaknesses – will allow you to become your best physician. Along with your own experience and the expertise you seek from others, it's vital to have the proper support, not only from your friends, family, and colleagues, but also from YOURSELF. No one else can make you follow through with these strategies.

Once you decide to actively make a change, you will be tested to see if you are serious. If everything were easy, there would be no point in learning from our day-to-day experiences. Take whatever comes your way as a lesson to push through and manifest your ultimate health goal as a reality. Things can go either way. You can let the massive stress of the pain and emotional frustration bring you down, or you can use this as fuel to get serious about what you deserve: your optimal wellbeing. Determination and consistency are all it takes, though easier said than done.

THE OTHER SIDE OF THE TUNNEL

When it seems as if there's no hope, no reason to go further, this is actually the best time to push through. Have you ever had to reschedule or put off obligations because of an episode? Yes, most likely. So, what did you do? Rested and healed, then, if possible, completed the obligation when you were able to, right? Same idea. If you're someone who gives up easily, this may be more of a challenge. Know you weren't put on this earth in vain. You had enough strength to enter this world and pave your way this far. It should only get better from here, unless you tell yourself that it will not. You are in control of your destiny. Remember that.

"The source of evil is in your body. Evil entices the body through temptation of its weakest virtue. There can be no divinity in the unclean temple where abomination rules."

– Ancient Egyptian proverb

Your cells need you to provide them with justice, or they will leave you to fight off what is sucking the joy out of your life.

The weakest virtue you have will be tested time and time again until you learn from it. To overcome challenges associated with sickle cell, we must be able to recognize our weakest virtue. If you're the type of person who gets easily frustrated or irritable, there may be situations that bring out these emotions to the surface. We should learn from the way we recognize and respond to such events, or they can drag us further into disappointment and illness. Once you identify your weakest virtues, you may naturally want to avoid situations that throw that weakness right in your face. This is an important clue to learning what stops you from moving forward. Developing your healthcare plan and maintaining your best health begins with you.

Chapter 12
Your Ultimate Plan

Living with sickle cell has had a great impact on my character and my life. I have been through instances when I've wondered how I would survive the pain because it can be so excruciating. Instances where I've fallen into a "conscious coma" have been terrifying. I refer to them as conscious comas because, even though I'm conscious, I cannot function with my own effort. While my body is in pain, not allowing me to move, my mind is thrown into the darkness of the abyss, away from this world and my usual perspective of it. I am left truly distant and in darkness.

I have gained additional strength and courage through these toughest of times. When my mind slips back into complete consciousness, I can then deeply feel why I need to continue my work here on earth. Experiencing both extremes – the void of desolation and the blessings of life – makes me realize how fortunate we are to be alive. This has only intensified my passion for others to experience what vitality should really feel like.

Sickle cell can force us to become the person we need to be in order to weather the storm. An attitude of acceptance will guide your decisions toward positive outcomes. To reduce the stress and concerns associated with this condition, consistency is key. Take it one step, one day at a time, with the techniques that resonate with you.

Oxygenating your body with foods, liquids, exercise, mindfulness, and deep breathing will enhance the functioning of red blood cells. Pay attention to the specifics of your organ systems and identify your weak points to improve your overall health. Specific non-invasive evaluations will help reveal items within your body that may cause decreased functioning of red blood cells. An individualized meal plan will address your own particular needs and requirements.

The thoughts you focus on consistently will eventually manifest and alter the frequency of your cells. Be careful what you think and wish for; you may actually get it! Methods such as cryotherapy, massage therapy, and flotation assist in improving blood flow and relieving muscle tension. Tracking your progress is essential; you will know if what you are doing is keeping you on the right track or moving you further from your healing. Many obstacles are faced when making changes to your health. It's important to remember why you are doing this and keep the bigger picture in mind.

Here you are. You've implemented vital steps towards greater health. Your cells have been reaping the benefits and, in turn, have been the very force in fueling your wellness. What differences have you noticed in your journey? Go back to the first entry in your tracking sheet and see where you've come from. If you truly take this seriously and make it a priority to encourage your body to heal itself in multiple ways, it must become a way of life.

With the support of an effective healthcare plan, including both conventional medicine and functional nutrition, you will slowly notice a decreased dependence on your medical team. Your personalized healthcare plan will provide you with the strength and confidence needed to move forward. All journeys begin with a single step. That single step for you is not only owning your circumstance but owning the power within you to change the frequencies inside your amazing body.

If you try, you will fail. The very act of *trying* anything tells your brain that there's plenty of room for disappointment. There is already an expectation of failure. Rather than *trying*, you must simply *do* it. Follow these essential steps slowly, one at a time, at your own pace. Doing everything at once is neither realistic nor sustainable. You want these great habits to stick.

INFLUENCE YOUR GENES

By reading this book and opening your mind to these new truths, hopefully, your relationship with sickle cell has been altered in some positive ways. You've gained new insight into how the mechanisms of your body function and react to outside influences.

As Stephen Covey puts it:

"You're not a product of your nature, that is, your genetic makeup, or your nurture, the things that have happened to you. Certainly, those things affect you powerfully, but they do not determine you."

If you want to do yourself a favor, be as practical as possible without being swayed by negative influences. A whole new perspective will awaken your enthusiasm for life.

We know that sickle cell is a genetic condition, but we do not need to be entirely at the mercy of our genes. We can influence our genes in various ways through our lifestyle decisions, habits, and health choices. This is what you bring to the table of your life. You are already able to make a difference because you are ready and willing to do so. You are the only one living in your precious temple. I'm sure you would agree that it deserves your nurturing in the best ways possible.

To do this, we all need support and guidance, especially through the most challenging circumstances when we may not think we have any control, but we do. In dealing with this condition, the goal is to evolve from the lowest point you can remember to becoming the vibrant being you were born to be. Incorporating as many steps as you can on your own is helpful, and seeking additional support may be positively life-changing. Take the time and care to select your healthcare team to assist in your healing journey, so you can be confident in the quality of care you receive.

Assisting individuals with sickle cell anemia in my practice has significantly enhanced my understanding of the causes and effects of symptoms associated with this condition. The steps outlined in these pages have been tremendously helpful. We all manifest symptoms differently, so having additional guidance can constructively transform your everyday life. I encourage you to question all aspects of your transition towards greater health by knowing your own patterns, strengths, and weaknesses. Becoming aware of your options and putting them into practice will enhance your understanding and progress of your individual journey.

Taking time out for your health is essential. The additional guidance of someone who can truly relate to you is equally important. By utilizing what has worked, this framework is designed to help you gain back your strength, energy, and cellular vitality.

When these strategies are put into practice, the very joy of life resurfaces, allowing us to become our own health creators. By becoming the source of your own joy and being grateful for what sickle cell has revealed, finding ways to make positive shifts in your current relationship with what is a part of you may become easier. Resisting yourself can only push you away from your goals. Becoming one with your emotions and relationship with sickle cell will make your efforts more meaningful and successful.

Your efforts to rejuvenate your cells shouldn't stop when you are pain-free, just like breathing doesn't stop when you're not focusing on it. Your life is ongoing. Therefore, your efforts should be focused on making your internal processes as efficient as possible. Providing for yourself will become more joyous and less stressful with your unique, individualized plan in place. Above all, I am rooting for you to implement these steps so that you can be more present for yourself, your responsibilities, and your family.

As you continue your health journey, I would love to hear from you about your successes and challenges. Together, we can build a genuine support system.

"I cannot believe that the purpose of life is to be happy. I think the purpose of life is to be useful, to be responsible, to be compassionate. It is, above all, to matter: to count, to stand for something, to have made some difference that you have lived at all."

– Leo C. Rosten.

Reflection Pages: Your Path to Victory

This section is designed to help you reflect, personalize, and put into practice what you've learned throughout this book. Take a quiet moment, breathe deeply, and write from the heart. Your words hold power — they plant the seeds of transformation.

MY WELLNESS COMMITMENTS

These commitments are your sacred agreement with your body, mind, and spirit.

What promises will you make to yourself as you begin (or continue) your healing journey?

I commit to:

1. ___________________________________

2. ___________________________________

3. ___________________________________

THREE CHANGES I WILL MAKE TO SUPPORT MY HEALTH

Small, consistent actions lead to lasting transformation.

What shifts will help you align more deeply with vitality, peace, and strength?

1. ____

2. ____

3. ____

AFFIRMATIONS FOR MY HEALING JOURNEY

Affirmations reprogram the subconscious mind for healing and resilience.

Write a few affirmations that speak directly to your journey:

1. ____

2. ____

3. ____

MY HEALING VISION

Every great transformation begins with a vision — a clear picture of the life you are creating. Take a moment to imagine yourself living in radiant health, peace, and joy.

What does that look and feel like for you?

Use this space to describe your vision in as much detail as you can:

- How does your body feel?

- What brings you joy and energy each day?

- How do you nourish yourself — physically, emotionally, and spiritually?

- Who are you becoming as you continue to heal?

My Healing Vision:

<u>***Remember:***</u> The clearer your vision, the stronger your vibration. Every thought you nurture helps shape the reality you desire.

WHAT VICTORY MEANS TO ME

This is your space to define what *Victory* truly means in your own words.

Consider:

- What does living victoriously look like for me?

- What have I overcome?

- What am I proud of today?

- How do I want to celebrate my progress?

Victory, to me, is:

<u>**Note:**</u> Let your definition of Victory evolve as you do. Each chapter of your life reveals new layers of strength and wisdom.

****

Take a moment to thank yourself for showing up — for reading, reflecting, and choosing wellness.

Each step you take brings you closer to your own victory.